Oxford Handbook of
Medical
Imaging

Edited by

Michael J. Darby

Consultant Radiologist
Leeds Teaching Hospitals NHS Trust
Leeds, UK

Dominic A. Barron

Consultant Radiologist
Leeds Teaching Hospitals NHS Trust
Leeds, UK

Rachel E. Hyland

Consultant Radiologist
Leeds Teaching Hospitals NHS Trust
Leeds, UK

OXFORD
UNIVERSITY PRESS

OXFORD
UNIVERSITY PRESS

Great Clarendon Street, Oxford OX2 6DP

Oxford University Press is a department of the University of Oxford.
It furthers the University's objective of excellence in research, scholarship,
and education by publishing worldwide in

Oxford New York

Auckland Cape Town Dar es Salaam Hong Kong Karachi
Kuala Lumpur Madrid Melbourne Mexico City Nairobi
New Delhi Shanghai Taipei Toronto

With offices in

Argentina Austria Brazil Chile Czech Republic France Greece
Guatemala Hungary Italy Japan Poland Portugal Singapore
South Korea Switzerland Thailand Turkey Ukraine Vietnam

Oxford is a registered trade mark of Oxford University Press
in the UK and in certain other countries

Published in the United States
by Oxford University Press Inc., New York

© Oxford University Press, 2012

British Library Cataloguing in Publication Data
Data available

Library of Congress Cataloguing-in-Publication Data
Darby, Michael (Michael J.)
  Oxford handbook of medical imaging/Michael Darby, Dominic Barron,
  Rachel Hyland.
      p. ; cm.—(Oxford handbooks)
  Handbook of medical imaging
  Includes index.
  ISBN 978–0–19–921636–9 (alk. paper)
  I. Barron, Dominic. II. Hyland, Rachel. III. Title. IV. Title:
  Handbook of medical imaging. V. Series: Oxford handbooks.
  [DNLM: 1. Diagnostic Imaging—Handbooks. WN 39]
  LC classification not assigned
  616.07'57—dc23   2011033024

Typeset by Cenveo, Bangalore, India
Printed in China
on acid-free paper through
Asia Pacific Offset

ISBN 978–0–19–921636–9

10 9 8 7 6 5 4 3 2 1

Preface

Radiology is becoming more and more important in the initial diagnosis, follow up, and, increasingly, the treatment of patients. At the same time it becomes more complex, and covers every anatomical and organ system group.

This book is written using a system-based approach, covering the various modalities and explaining their relevance in each situation. For each system there are three separate sections. The first deals with common presenting symptoms, listing the most likely diagnoses. There is then a review of the imaging approach to each of these presenting conditions and the value of each modality. The second section lists the common radiological findings which may be encountered and the differential diagnoses which need to be considered. The final section discusses in detail a number of common conditions.

Using this approach, the authors hope that this book will help to guide junior doctors and other professionals through the increasingly varied roles imaging can play in the management of their patients.

With a book of this size, it is impossible to include all known conditions. The authors have concentrated on those conditions which are either common, or of such importance that any delay in diagnosis may be significant.

The authors would value feedback on the text which could lead to improvements being made in future editions.

Acknowledgements

In preparing the text, the authors are aware that many of the lists, statistics used, and radiological signs described have previously been published. Acknowledgement is made to the following texts:

Chapman S. Nakielny R. *Aids to Radiological Differential Diagnosis*, 5th edition. Philadelphia: WB Saunders, 2009.

Dähnert W. *Radiology Review Manual*, 7th revised international edition. Baltimore: Lippincott Williams & Wilkins, 2011.

Contents

Contributors

Raneem Albazaz
SpR Leeds
Bradford Radiology Training
Scheme, UK

Anu Balan
Consultant Radiologist
Addenbrookes Hospital
Cambridge University Hospitals
NHS Foundation Trust
Cambridge, UK

Priya Bhatnagar
Leeds Teaching Hospitals NHS
Trust, Leeds, UK

Robert Briggs
Consultant Radiologist
Calderdale and Huddersfield
NHS Foundation Trust, UK

Barbara Dall
Consultant Breast Radiologist
Leeds Teaching Hospitals
NHS Trust
Leeds, UK

Karen Flood
SpR Leeds
Bradford Radiology Training
Scheme, UK

Nerys Forrester
SpR Leeds
Bradford Radiology Training
Scheme, UK

Shishir Karthik
SpR Leeds
Bradford Radiology Training
Scheme, UK

Amit Lakkaraju
Musculoskeletal Radiology Fellow
Royal Liverpool Hospital
Prescott St, Liverpool, UK

Nalinda Panditaratne
SpR Leeds
Bradford Radiology Training
Scheme, UK

Sabrina Rajan
SpR Leeds
Bradford Radiology Training
Scheme, UK

Emma Rowbotham
SpR Leeds
Bradford Radiology Training
Scheme, UK

Nisha Sharma
Director of Breast Screening
Leeds/Wakefield Breast
Screening unit, UK

Stephen Slater
SpR Leeds
Bradford Radiology Training
Scheme, UK

Gemma Smith
Consultant Radiologist
Bradford Teaching Hospitals NHS
Foundation Trust, UK

Manil Subesinghe
SpR Leeds
Bradford Radiology Training
Scheme, UK

Sophie Swinson
SpR Leeds
Bradford Radiology Training
Scheme, UK

Stuart Viner
Consultant Radiologist
Bradford Teaching Hospitals NHS
Foundation Trust, UK

Symbols and abbreviations

📖	cross-reference
≈	approximately
±	with or without
α	alpha
β	beta
γ	gamma
2D	2-dimensional
3D	3-dimensional
ABG	arterial blood gases
ACE	angiotensin converting enzyme
AP	anteroposterior
AS	aortic stenosis
ASD	atrial septal defect
ATN	acute tubular necrosis
AV	arteriovenous
AVF	arteriovenous fistula
AVM	arteriovenous malformation
AVN	avascular necrosis
BSO	bilateral salpingo-oophorectomy
Ca	calcium
CC	craniocaudal
CEA	carcinoembryonic antigen
CM	cardiomyopathy
CMCJ	carpometacarpal joint
COPD	chronic obstructive pulmonary disease
CRP	C-reactive protein
CT	computed tomography
CTA	computed tomography angiography
CTPA	computed tomography pulmonary angiography
CTU	CT urogram
CXR	chest X-ray
DCBE	double-contrast barium enema
DCM	dilated cardiomyopathy
DIPJ	distal interphalangeal joint
DMSA	dimercaptosuccinic acid
DRE	digital rectal examination

DTPA	diethylene triamine pentaacetic acid
DVT	deep vein thrombosis
DWI	diffusion-weighted imaging
EAA	extrinsic allergic alveolitis
ECG	electrocardiogram
EF	ejection fraction
e.g.	for example
ERCP	endoscopic retrograde cholangiopancreatography
ESR	erythrocyte sedimentation rate
EUS	endoscopic ultrasound
FAST	focused assessment with sonography for trauma *or* face arm speech test
Fbc	full blood count
FDG	fluorodeoxy-D-glucose
FIGO	International Federation of Gynaecology and Obstetrics
FLAIR	fluid attenuated inversion recovery
GCS	Glasgow Coma Score
GCT	germ cell tumour
GI	gastrointestinal
GU	genitourinary
HCC	hepatocellular carcinoma
HCG	human chorionic gonadotropin
HCM	hypertrophic cardiomyopathy
HPT	hyperparathyroidism
HRCT	high resolution computed tomography
HRT	hormone replacement therapy
HU	Hounsfield unit
IMB	intermenstrual bleeding
INR	international normalized ratio
IV	intravenous
IVC	inferior vena cava
IVU	intravenous urogram
JVP	jugular venous pressure
keV	kilo-electron volts
KUB	kidneys, ureters, bladder
LBO	large-bowel obstruction
LFT	liver function tests
LMP	last menstrual period
LN	lymph node
LVF	left ventricular failure

ml	millilitre/s
mg	milligram/s
m/s	metres per second
MAG3	mercapto acetyl triglycerine
MC&S	microscopy, culture, and sensitivity
MCPJ	metacarpophalangeal joint
MCUG	micturating cystourethrogram
MDP	methyl-di-phosphonate
Mg	magnesium
MHz	megahertz
MI	myocardial infarction
MIBG	metaiodobenzylguanidine
MLO	mediolateral oblique
MR	magnetic resonance or mitral regurgitation
MRCP	magnetic resonance cholangiopancreatography
MRE	magnetic resonance enterography
MRI	magnetic resonance tomography
MS	mitral stenosis
mSv	millisievert
NCCT	non-contrast computed tomography
NG	nasogastric
NICE	National Institute for Health and Clinical Excellence
NJ	nasojejunal
NSAID	non-steroidal anti-inflammatory
OGD	oesophagogastroduodenoscopy
OHCM	*Oxford Handbook of Clinical Medicine*, eighth edition (2010)
PA	posteroanterior
PACS	picture archive communication systems
PCD	peripheral vascular disease
PCI	primary percutaneous intervention
PDA	patent ductus arteriosus
PET	positron emission tomography
PIPJ	proximal interphalangeal joint
PMB	postmenopausal bleeding
PMF	progressive massive fibrosis
PSA	prostate specific antigen
RCM	restrictive cardiomyopathy
RTA	road traffic accident
SAH	subarachnoid haemorrhage
SBFT	small bowel follow through

SLE	systemic lupus erythematosus
SPECT	single-photon emission computed tomography
SSRI	selective serotonin reuptake inhibitor
SUV	standardized uptake value
TA	transabdominal
TB	tuberculosis
Tc	technetium
TCC	transitional cell cancer
TMN	tumour, node, metastasis
TOE	transoesophageal echocardiography
TRUS	transrectal ultrasound
TURP	transurethral resection prostate
TV	transvaginal
U&E	urea and electrolytes
UC	ulcerative colitis
Uro	urological
UTI	urinary tract infection
VQ	ventilation/perfusion
VSD	ventricular septal defect
WCC	white cell count

Techniques

Plain film radiography

The electromagnetic spectrum is comprised of different types of radiation, which all travel at the same velocity in a vacuum, 3×10^8 m/s (speed of light), but which vary in their frequency, wavelength, and energy. Plain film radiography utilizes X-rays, which are a type of ionizing radiation owing to their extremely short wavelengths and high energies.

Using X-ray tubes, electrons produced by thermionic emission from the negatively charged cathode are accelerated towards the positively charged anode. These fast moving electrons interact with the atoms of the metallic anode and by doing so their kinetic energy is converted into X-rays (1%) and thermal energy (99%). Most diagnostic radiology sets have anodes made of a tungsten–rhenium alloy but in mammography either molybdenum or rhenium is used.

X-rays that travel through the tissues of the body can be absorbed or scattered. Both these processes contribute to attenuation of the primary X-ray beam. X-rays that are transmitted through the patient reflect a varying degree of attenuation, which is dependent upon several factors including the atomic numbers and physical densities of the materials traversed in addition to the initial energies of the incident primary X-ray beam.

The final radiographic image is formed entirely of transmitted X-rays. Until very recently, radiographic film was used to display the final image. X-rays that have passed through air are minimally attenuated and therefore maximally transmitted, causing film blackening. X-rays that have passed through bone are heavily attenuated with very few transmitted, resulting in minimal film exposure and a resultant white appearance.

Most modern radiology departments now use digital radiographic acquisition in conjunction with picture archiving communication systems (PACS). Digital image plates replace radiographic film with computers playing a fundamental role in post-processing and storage. The final image is then displayed on a dedicated viewing monitor.

Although plain film radiography utilizes ionizing X-ray radiation, the effective doses for the majority of examinations performed are low in comparison to computed tomography (CT). It is cheap, readily accessible, and easy to perform and for these reasons is commonly the first-line imaging modality utilized by clinicians.

The main applications of plain radiography are initial investigation of the thorax, abdomen, and skeletal system, in particular trauma and joint-based disease (Fig. 1.1). Despite its high spatial resolution, the major disadvantage of radiography is its poor soft tissue contrast resolution, which is where other modalities such as magnetic resonance imaging (MRI) and CT, to a lesser extent, are more useful.

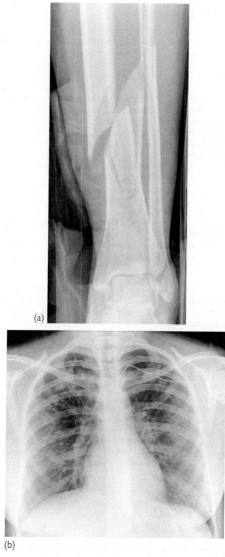

Fig. 1.1 a) AP radiograph of the ankle joint demonstrating a multisegmental fracture of the distal tibia and fibula. b) Chest radiograph demonstrating generalized patchy shadowing throughout both lungs and a central line in a 20-year-old with cystic fibrosis.

Fluoroscopy

Historically the first mode of medical imaging to use ionizing radiation, dating back to 1895. The patient was placed between an X-ray source and the observing radiologist looked down a tube with a fluoroscopic coating, unfortunately with substantial radiation to the radiologist. Thankfully monitors were introduced to display images obtained by intensifier units. Fluoroscopy uses rapid pulses or streams of X-rays to produce a real-time image rather like a moving radiograph. The devices can be angled or moved in 3 dimensions to achieve optimal views to demonstrate pathology.

Fluoroscopy has a role in both diagnostic and procedural work, including vascular intervention and use in operating theatres. Orthopaedics use screening to align fixation plates and reduce fractures. Musculoskeletal (MSK) radiologists use it to perform arthrograms and injections. Gastrointestinal (GI) and urological (Uro) radiologists use screening (see 'Imaging').

Contrast agents are central to GI and Uro radiology fluoroscopy:
- Positive agents such as barium and iodine block X-rays; pathology often appears as a filling defect within the contrast.
- Negative agents (air and water) distend structures/lumens and allow more X-rays through.
- Double-contrast techniques utilize both of the above and allow surfaces to be visualized in detail (Fig. 1.2), e.g. bowel mucosa.

Imaging

Visualization of the GI tract lends itself well to fluoroscopy. Luminal contrast can be administered either orally or per rectum. Care is required in preparing the patient correctly; fasting or bowel laxative preparation may be required. Check local protocols for each study.

GI radiology
- Swallow: pharynx and oesophagus.
- Meal: lower oesophagus, stomach, and duodenal cap.
- Small bowel meal: small bowel, in particular the terminal ileum.
- Single-contrast water soluble upper or lower GI study: to identify perforation or obstruction especially useful postoperatively.
- Double-contrast enema: colonic pathology, excellent mucosal detail caution not in acute colitis or diverticulitis (perforation risk).
- Biliary imaging, including endoscopic retrograde cholangiopancreatography (ERCP).
- Procedures: nasogastric (NG) and nasojejunal (NJ) tube placement. Oesophageal and colonic stents.

Uro radiology
- Nephrostomy insertion.
- Nephrostogram.
- Ureteric stent insertion.
- Cystogram, urethrogram.
- Retrograde ureterograms (performed in theatre by urologists).
- Loopograms or conduitograms (postoperative studies performed by retrograde administration of contrast into a neo-bladder after urinary diversions surgery to examine both the conduit and upper tracts).

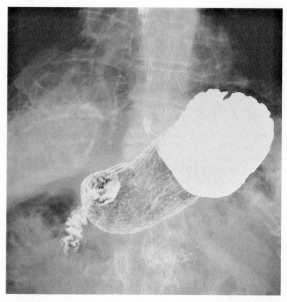

Fig. 1.2 Image from an upper GI contrast study, showing the double-contrast effect of the radio-opaque barium, against the radiolucent air. The stomach folds can be clearly seen in the distal stomach.

Angiography

Angiography is an imaging technique where a radio-opaque contrast agent is injected intravenously or intra-arterially and the target vessel is visualized using fluoroscopy. The image thus acquired is called an angiogram. Visceral, peripheral, and central arteries and veins can be imaged depending on the indication (Fig. 1.3).

Indications

Angiography can identify:
- Site of vascular stenosis or occlusion.
- Vascular anatomy or anomalies prior to intervention or surgery.
- Active bleeding.
- Arterial dissection.
- Graft and transplant angiography.

Procedure

Access

The common femoral vein or artery is most commonly used. The brachial route is an alternative, used when the femoral approach is either inappropriate (e.g. demonstration of upper limb venous anatomy prior to fistula formation) or unavailable.

Rarely, direct puncture of a graft site may be performed.

Jugular or subclavian vein puncture may also be performed, if the superior (SVC) or inferior vena cava (IVC) needs to be visualized.

Local preparation

The site is cleaned and under strict asepsis the appropriate vessel is targeted after administering local anaesthesia.

Technique

The choice of proper equipment prior to beginning the procedure is vital to its success.

The vessel may be punctured using anatomical landmarks, but in some cases either ultrasound or fluoroscopic guidance is needed.

Once the vessel is punctured, a guidewire is passed and its position confirmed with fluoroscopy. An appropriate vascular catheter is passed over the guidewire, which is then removed.

Contrast is then either hand injected (if a small peripheral artery or vein is to be visualized) or pump injected (if aorta or IVC is to be visualized) and the anatomy is demonstrated.

If necessary the appropriate vascular bed may then be selectively catheterized using special catheters or micro-catheters.

Once the diagnostic images are acquired, these can then be transferred to an adjacent screen to be used as a road map for further intervention.

Contrast agents

The commonest agents are iodine-based compounds of different types. Hyperosmolar and ionic agents are not commonly used today, as iso-osmolar or hypo-osmolar non-ionic agents are preferred.

Carbon dioxide is used as a negative contrast agent for angiography in patients with iodine allergy or renal failure. Gadolinium is also an alternative to iodinated agents.

Complications

- Puncture site complications: haematoma, pseudo-aneurysm, arteriovenous (AV) fistula and infection.
- Contrast allergy and anaphylaxis.
- Trauma to the vessel, leading to dissection, rupture, bleeding, or occlusion.

Alternatives to conventional angiography

With the development of both CT and MR, the diagnostic role of invasive angiography is diminishing. Contrast-enhanced CT angiography and both contrast enhanced and unenhanced MR (such as time of flight and phase contrast MR) can be used to visualize different vascular beds for diagnostic purposes. These can then be used to guide conventional angiographic intervention.

Useful information for the radiologist

It is important to know about the patient's renal function, clotting profile, and any major underlying morbidity as often these patients need to lie flat for long periods of time.

Prior imaging and background clinical history may provide useful information of the exact vascular bed to be imaged.

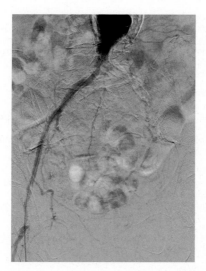

Fig. 1.3 Coronal image from an angiography study in a patient with peripheral vascular disease who presented with an acutely ischaemic left leg. The angiogram shows an occluded left iliac system, and heavily calcified right iliac arteries.

Ultrasound

Ultrasound imaging (Fig. 1.4) uses high-frequency sound waves (1–20MHz) and the way they travel through tissues, to image different areas of the body. Tissues of different densities reflect the sound waves back to the probe with their own characteristics. These variances are used to generate an image.

- Ultrasoundwaves are reflected by bone and gas. It is therefore poor for imaging these bodily tissues and structures containing gas.
- It is an operator-dependant form of imaging that is the first line of investigation in biliary, cardiac, renal, obstetric, and many vascular diseases.
- It is frequently used to perform guided aspiration, biopsies, and insertion of drains (thoracic or abdomino-pelvic).
- The use of Doppler ultrasound allows assessment of patency and flow in blood vessels.

Abdominal scan

This investigation involves the evaluation of the solid organs of the abdomen (liver, gallbladder, pancreas, aorta, kidneys, spleen).
It is used to assess:

- Liver size and texture, assessment of any potential masses.
- Biliary system: biliary duct dilatation, presence of stones, and gallbladder wall thickness.
- Doppler of hepatic artery/veins and portal vein for flow characteristics.
- Pancreas.
- Aorta: assessing diameter for presence of an aneurysm.
- Kidneys: for size, texture, presence of calculi and size of collecting system (i.e. looking for hydronephrosis). The bladder is not routinely examined in an abdominal ultrasound scan, therefore a dedicated renal examination should be requested if this is required.
- Spleen: size and texture.

Urinary tract scan

Assessment of kidneys (Fig. 1.5) and bladder:

- Examination is performed with a full bladder to assess the bladder wall thickness accurately.
- Pre- and post-micturition imaging can be obtained to gain information about the bladder capacity and emptying.

Pelvic scan

Assessment of the uterus, ovaries, and pregnancy. Scans can be performed:

- Transabdominally (TA): patient must have a full bladder.
- Transvaginally (TV): this gives a more detailed assessment of the gynaecological organs.

Testicular scan

This is used to assess testicular masses such as:

- Tumours.
- Hydrocoeles.
- Inflammation/infection.

Neck

Ultrasound is used to assess:
- Neck and thyroid masses.
- Presence and characteristics of lymph nodes.

Cardiac ultrasound

Measurement of chamber size. Accurate assessment of valve and wall motion:
- 2D echocardiography provides real-time images of the anatomy and spatial relationships.
- Duplex Doppler includes colour coding of flow directions and allows direct visualization of shunts and regurgitant flow.

Vascular scan

Assessment of:
- Carotid artery disease.
- Peripheral vasculature.
- Venous imaging.

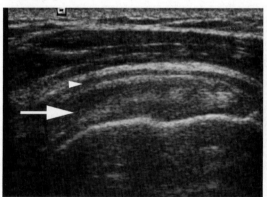

Fig. 1.4 Longitudinal scan of the shoulder rotator cuff in a patient with restricted shoulder movements. The arrow points to the supraspinatus tendon and the arrowhead to the thickened subacromial bursa consistent with subacromial bursitis.

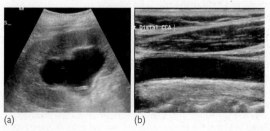

(a) (b)

Fig. 1.5 a) Longitudinal image of a kidney with a dilated collecting system consistent with hydronephrosis. b) Longitudinal image of the common carotid artery with crosses outlining the tunica intima.

Computed tomography

Computed tomography (CT) uses X-rays to produce cross-sectional images of the body (Fig. 1.6). Images are generated by rotation of an X-ray tube around the patient. A ring of detectors located around the patient then measures the transmitted radiation. The numerical data obtained is computer processed to reconstruct the final images.

In spiral or helical scanners the X-ray tube rotates continuously around the patient whilst the table, on which the patient is lying, is mechanically moved through the X-ray beam. This allows a continuous volume of data to be obtained rather than acquiring data one slice at a time. All modern CT scanners utilize spiral scanning and incorporate multiple rows of detector rings (known as multislice or multidetector scanners). Multidetector spiral CT has a number of advantages over single slice scanning:

- Faster scanning: a greater area of the patient can be covered in a given time by the X-ray beam.
- Better dynamic imaging: as a consequence of faster scanning, it is possible to acquire images during different phases of passage of contrast through tissues of interest.
- Thinner slices: thin slices, down to sub-millimetre thickness, can be acquired thereby improving spatial resolution.
- Genuine 3D imaging: this requires thin slices with equal x/y/z dimensions. This allows the volume of data to be reformatted in various planes (axial, sagittal, coronal, oblique) and as 3D representations of structures.

CT image reconstruction

Every CT slice is subdivided into a matrix of up to 1024 x 1024 volume elements (voxels). Each voxel has been traversed during the scan by numerous X-ray photos and the intensity of the transmitted radiation measured by detectors. From these intensity readings, the density or attenuation value of the tissue at each point in the slice can be calculated. The viewed image is then reconstructed as a corresponding matrix of picture elements (pixels).

Hounsfield unit or CT number

Each pixel is assigned a numerical value, which is the average of all the attenuation values contained within the corresponding voxel. This number is compared to the attenuation value of water and displayed on a scale of arbitrary units known as the Hounsfield unit (HU) or CT number (named after Sir Godfrey Hounsfield who developed the first CT scanner in 1972).

This scale assigns water an attenuation value of zero HU. The range of CT numbers is usually 2000HU. Each number represents a shade of grey with +1000 (white) and −1000 (black) at either end of the spectrum.

Window level and window width

The range of CT numbers recognized by the computer is 2000, but the human eye can only distinguish 11 different shades of grey. Hence, in order to be able to interpret the image, only a limited number of HU are displayed. This is achieved by setting the window level and window width on the computer to a suitable range of HU, depending on the tissue being studied.

The term window level represents the central HU of all the numbers within the window width.

The window width covers the HU of all the tissues of interest, which are displayed as various shades of grey. Tissues with HU outside this range are displayed as either black or white.

Contrast media

Contrast between the tissues of the body can be improved by the use of contrast agents. These are usually substances with high molecular weight, which increase the attenuation value of tissues they opacify.

Oral contrast

This is used to opacify bowel thereby making it easier to identify pathology. Iodine-based preparations are usually used and are normally given to the patient to drink 1 hour prior to the examination.

Intravenous contrast

Iodine-based preparations are usually used to opacify the vascular tree. Different phases of enhancement can be obtained, depending on the timing of image acquisition. IV contrast is used to differentiate normal blood vessels from abnormal masses and to demonstrate the vascular nature of an abnormality.

Drawbacks of CT

These include the use of ionizing radiation (doses vary according to the type of examination but can be high), hazards of IV contrast (renal impairment, allergy), lack of portability, and relative cost. Some areas of the body are imaged poorly with CT, including the posterior cranial fossa and spine.

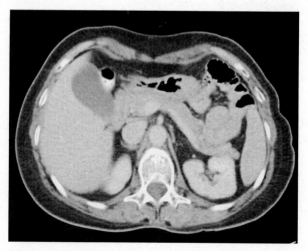

Fig. 1.6 Axial CT image showing normal upper abdominal anatomy.

Nuclear medicine (traditional)

Description

Nuclear medicine differs from other forms of imaging in that it shows the physiological function of a system rather than an anatomical region. Radioactive isotopes permit detection by emitting gamma radiation (γ) which is detected by a gamma camera. In most cases the radioisotope is coupled to a biologically active molecule or drug to localize to a desired system. Pathological conditions may lead to increased uptake, i.e. hotspots or decreased activity, i.e. cold spots.

Radionuclides and radiopharmaceuticals

When a radioactive substance decays it may emit radiation in the form of alpha (α) and beta (β) particles and electromagnetic radiation in the form of gamma rays and X-rays. It is gamma rays, which penetrate the body allowing detection, which are exploited in nuclear medicine imaging. Radionuclides are selected which produce a high volume of gamma emissions without emitting harmful particulate radiation (i.e. α or β particles). The half-life needs to be only long enough for the intended use, usually a few hours.

The radionuclide is manufactured artificially and degrades spontaneously. The commonest radionuclide in use is technetium 99m (Tc-99m). This decays to technetium 99 with the emission of a γ ray of 140keV (kilo-electron volts) and has a half-life of 6 hours.

When a radionuclide is coupled with a drug, it is called a radiopharmaceutical. The pharmaceutical is chosen to rapidly localize to the intended target without side effects. Certain radionuclides, e.g. I-123 and Ga-67, localize to the desired area without an attached pharmaceutical. The radiopharmaceutical is injected, ingested orally, or inhaled.

The gamma camera

The gamma camera consists of a large sodium iodide crystal with thallium iodide as an activator. The gamma rays striking the camera are converted into light photons, which are multiplied and converted into small voltage pulses to record activity. Some scattered rays are absorbed by a collimator placed in front of the crystal and the pulse height analyser selects photons of a predetermined narrow spectrum. The whole field image is shown on a cathode ray tube, which can be photographed or captured as an electrical pulse for a digital image.

The image

The patient must sit or lie still in front of the gamma camera until sufficient activity is recorded. Images are acquired in each desired plane, e.g. anterior, posterior, lateral, or oblique. The image may be static or multiple frames may be acquired over a period of time to create dynamic images.

rt

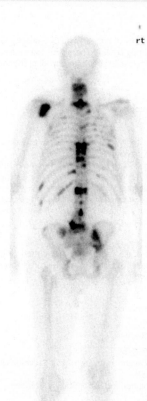

Fig. 1.7 Selected image from a technetium bone scan in a patient with prostate cancer. Multiple areas of increased radioisotope uptake are consistent with bony metastases.

Indications

There are multiple uses of nuclear medicine imaging. Some of the commonest types of imaging are listed here with common indications.

- Bone scan: Tc-99m labelled MDP (methyl-di-phosphonate):
  - Infection.
  - Occult fracture.
  - Bone metastases (Fig. 1.7).
- Myocardial perfusion scan: Tl-201 chloride.
- Thyroid uptake scan: I-123.
- Renal imaging:
  - Static imaging: Tc-99m DMSA (dimercaptosuccinic acid)—for split renal function, ?renal scars.
  - Dynamic imaging: Tc-99m DTPA (diethylene triamine penta-acetic acid) or Tc-99m MAG 3 (mercaptoacetyltriglycine)—renal excretion, renovascular hypertension.
- Ventilation/perfusion scan (V/Q scan): inhaled gas, e.g. Kr-81m or Tc-99m DTPA and injected Tc-99m albumin macroaggregates:
  - Pulmonary embolus exclusion (Fig. 1.8).

Contraindications

The radiation dose of each scan must be weighed up against the alternative imaging techniques available. Particular care is needed with children, pregnant women, and breastfeeding mothers.

Advantages

- Demonstrates physiology.
- Widely available.
- Relatively cheap.

Disadvantages

- Radiation dose. Patient continues to emit radiation after procedure, in diminishing doses.
- Poor spatial resolution for anatomical localization.
- Time-consuming.

Dose

The administered dose is measured in becquerels (usually in kilo- or mega-becquerels). The effective patient dose is given in millisievert (mSv).

The effective dose of a nuclear medicine scan varies with type and administered does of radiopharmaceutical. The effective dose of a typical Tc-99m MDP bone scan is 3mSv (compared to chest radiograph = 0.1mSv, average annual background radiation UK = 2.6mSv).

Patient preparation

Certain types of nuclear medicine scan require patient preparation in terms of fasting, stopping medication, or taking medication prior to the examination. It is worth checking local policy with your nuclear medicine scan team when requesting an investigation for your patient.

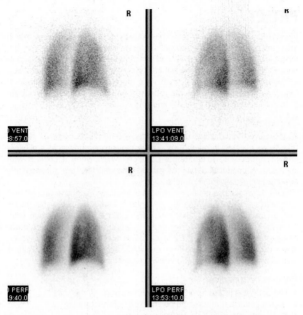

Fig. 1.8 Selected images from a V/Q scan, looking for a pulmonary embolus. Matched ventilation (upper row) and perfusion (lower row) in a normal scan.

PET-CT

PET-CT is a relatively new technique, rapidly developing a central role in many imaging pathways. It involves the fusion of images from two very different imaging modalities—positron emission tomography (PET) and computed tomography (CT). The patient undergoes both scans sequentially, in the same session, and the results are merged, giving a combination of functional information from the radioisotope PET scan and the accurate anatomical detail of CT (Figs. 1.9 and 1.10).

Technique

A short-lived radioactive tracer isotope—2–18 fluorodeoxy-D-glucose (FDG)—is injected intravenously. This radioisotope undergoes a process known as beta-decay, emitting a positron, which when it collides with an electron produces a pair of gamma photons that are subsequently detected within a gamma camera.

FDG is a glucose analogue that accumulates within areas of high intracellular metabolism and glycolysis. Tumour cells are highly metabolically active, and also retain FDG more than do normal cells, meaning that the isotope becomes concentrated within the tumour resulting in a 'hot spot' on the image. FDG is not cancer specific, however, and is taken up in all areas of high metabolic activity, such as the brain, as well as by areas of inflammation or increased muscle activity.

Patient preparation

- The patient is fasted for at least 4–6 hours prior to the scan.
- Plasma glucose levels should be checked before scanning.
- An IV injection of FDG is administered.
- The patient rests quietly for a period while the isotope circulates. Movement and talking are discouraged to prevent muscle uptake.
- Scanning begins approximately 60 minutes following the injection and the total scan time is approx. 30–90 minutes.
- Images are acquired from the top of the head to mid thighs, with the patient's arms above their head. Usually the CT is obtained first followed by the gamma camera images. Because the scanners are in the same gantry the patient remains on a single scanning table and in the same position during both scans.

Indications

- In general, PET is better than conventional imaging at demonstrating distant metastases from a wide variety of tumours. It is therefore used to complete the staging in cases where more traditional tests have suggested localized disease; e.g. in lung cancer, PET has been shown to upstage a significant proportion of patients thought on CT to be potentially operable.
- PET is being used to provide early assessment of tumour response to chemotherapy allowing regimens to be altered if appropriate.
- Also useful in early assessment of suspected disease recurrence in areas of post-treatment scarring or fibrosis.
- Research roles in assessing myocardial perfusion.
- Developing roles in neuro imaging.

Relative contraindications

- Pregnancy (high-dose examination, around 20mSv).
- Uncontrolled diabetes makes interpretation difficult.
- Patients must be able to lie still for considerable length of time.

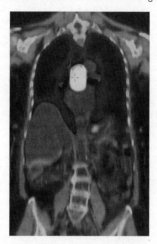

Fig. 1.9 Coronal image from staging PET-CT showing increased uptake of oesophageal tumour (calliper).

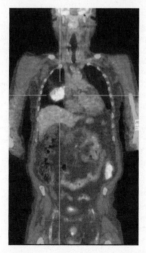

Fig. 1.10 Image from a staging PET scan in a patient with lung cancer. Second incidental focus found within the left flank, found to be an incidental colonic tumour. The other areas of increased uptake are physiological.

Magnetic resonance imaging

General principles

Materials placed in a magnetic field can absorb and then re-emit electromagnetic radiation of a specific frequency, usually in the form of radiosignals. When tissue is placed in a magnetic field (MRI scanner) the protons (hydrogen nuclei) align with the field. A radiofrequency electromagnetic field is then briefly turned on, causing the protons to alter their alignment relative to the field. When this field is turned off the protons return to the original magnetization alignment. These alignment changes create a signal which can be detected by the scanner. The frequency at which the protons resonate depends on the strength of the magnetic field. The position of protons in the body can be determined by applying additional magnetic fields during the scan, which allows an image of the body to be built up. These are created by turning gradient coils on and off which creates the knocking sounds heard during an MR scan.

Protons in different tissues return to their equilibrium state at different rates. By changing the parameters on the scanner, this effect is used to create contrast between different types of body tissue. Various sequences can be achieved by changing imaging parameters. Basic sequences are T1, T2, T2*, proton density, inversion recovery (short tau inversion recovery, STIR (Fig. 1.11); fluid attenuation inversion recovery, FLAIR). More specialized sequences include diffusion-weighted imaging (DWI), MR angiography and functional imaging. The most widely used MR contrast agents are gadolinium chelates. Gadolinium is a paramagnetic substance that enhances the relaxation rate of surrounding tissue thereby producing greater T1 signal i.e. 'bright' on T1 imaging.

Applications

MRI is used to image every part of the body, and is particularly useful for neurological conditions, disorders of the muscles and joints, tumours, and for showing abnormalities in the heart and blood vessels. While CT offers greater spatial resolution (ability to distinguish two structures a small distance apart as separate structures) MRI offers greater contrast resolution (ability to distinguish two similar, but not identical tissues).

MRI does not use ionizing radiation and there are as yet no reported long-term biological effects from prolonged exposure to a magnetic field. This makes MRI more appropriate in children and pregnancy.

There are disadvantages to MRI. Acquiring images is time consuming and scans can often last 20–40 minutes. Patients must be able to lie still for this length of time. Young children will often require a general anaesthetic. Patients with claustrophobia may not tolerate MRI and sedation or alternative imaging may be required.

Contraindications

There are absolute contraindications:
- Cardiac pacemakers.
- Cochlear implants.
- Tissue expanders.
- Ocular prostheses.

- Dental implants.
- Neurostimulators.
- Bone growth stimulators.
- Implantable cardiac defibrillators.
- Implantable drug infusion pumps.

New medical devices tend to be MRI compatible and MRI safe pacemakers are now available. Others to consider are orthopaedic implants/metalwork, vascular clips, intravascular coils and bullets/pellets/shrapnel. Most of these are safe, but they should be evaluated on a patient-by-patient basis. More information is freely available online (http://www.mrisafety.com).

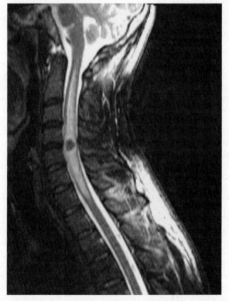

Fig. 1.11 Sagittal STIR image of the cervical spine showing intra-cord abscess and oedema secondary to tuberculosis.

Interventional radiology

Radiological interventional techniques use image guidance such as fluoroscopy, ultrasound, or CT to help in a diagnostic or therapeutic procedure. The role of interventional radiology is continually expanding and there is hardly any area of hospital medicine where it does not have an impact on patient management. The advantages include reduced risk as compared to surgery, shorter hospital stay, lower cost, greater comfort, quicker convalescence, and return to work.

Non-vascular intervention

Includes diagnostic biopsies, drainage of collections, GI procedures such as oesophageal, gastroduodenal and colonic stent placement, percutaneous gastrostomy and gastrojejunostomy insertions, biliary drainage, urological procedures such as percutaneous nephrostomy and antegrade ureteric stent placement, etc.

Vascular intervention

Includes procedures such as angiography (Fig. 1.12), angioplasty, stent placement, thrombolysis, EVAR (endovascular aneurysm repair), tumour embolization, uterine fibroid embolization, postpartum haemorrhage management, bronchial artery embolization, Hickman line insertions, Varicocoele embolization, IVC filter placement and retrieval, etc.

Pre-procedure preparation

- Confirm the clinical indication.
- Check previous imaging.
- Check the coagulation and infection screen as per local protocols.
- Consider use of medication such as sedatives, analgesics, etc.
- Choose the correct imaging modality for the procedure.
- Obtain informed consent.

Ultrasound-guided procedures

Ultrasound is used for various biopsy and drainage procedures. It is ideal if the target is clearly visible and a suitable approach is possible. The advantages of using ultrasound are that procedure is performed in real time, it can be done portably in ICU etc, and does not involve ionizing radiation.

The procedure can be performed using a needle guide attached to the ultrasound probe, which shows the path the needle will take. Another method is to use a freehand technique wherein the probe is fixed with one hand and the needle is advanced into the target with the other. The latter technique is more difficult and requires expertise.

CT-guided intervention

When it is not possible to access the target using ultrasound guidance (e.g. pathology within lung, related to bowel, etc.), CT guidance may be used. The puncture site is marked following a reference scan. Needle path to the target is planned. After each needle pass, the patient goes into the scanner and is then brought out again making the procedure more 'stop/start' and time consuming than when using US. Once the needle is in a satisfactory position, the appropriate procedure is performed.

Aftercare

This varies with the type of procedure, the general condition of patient, the coagulation status, etc. Depending on local protocols the procedure may be performed as a daycase and all aftercare takes place in the radiology department, or the patient may be returned to a ward in which case a written aftercare plan should go with them. It should always be mentioned if the procedure was difficult or if there were any immediate complications.

Complications

These vary with the type and site of procedure, and between individual patients. Serious complications are rare. Following are some of the important complications to look out for:

- Bleeding.
- Infection.
- Bowel perforation.
- Pneumothorax.

Most complications can be managed adequately but need to be thought about and recognized early.

Useful information for the radiologist

Detailed clinical history and clinical differential diagnosis, coagulation status, and infection screen. If the patient is uncooperative or extremely anxious then may need to consider pre-medications or sedation.

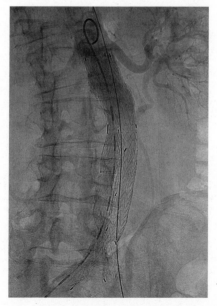

Fig. 1.12 Image from a vascular angiography study in a patient who has undergone endovascular repair of their abdominal aortic aneurysm. The stents can be clearly seen.

Respiratory differential diagnosis

Focal consolidation

- Pneumonia.
- Haemorrhage.
- Contusion.
- Alveolar cell carcinoma.
- Cryptogenic organizing pneumonia.
- Lymphoma.

Widespread consolidation

- Infection.
- Oedema.
- Pulmonary haemorrhage.
- Tumour:
  - BAC.
  - Lymphoma.
  - Widespread metastases.
- Proteinosis.
- Alveolitis.
- Cryptogenic organizing pneumonia.
- Eosinophilic pneumonia.

White out

- Mediastinum shifted toward white out:
  - Collapsed lung.
  - Pneumonectomy.
- Mediastinum shifted away from white out:
  - Pleural fluid.
  - Large mass.
- Mediastinum central:
  - Combination of collapse and fluid.
  - Widespread consolidation.
  - Pleural tumour.

Solitary lung mass

- Primary lung cancer.
- Solitary metastasis.
- Lymphoma.
- Benign tumour:
  - Carcinoid.
  - Hamartoma.
- Arteriovenous malformation (AVM).
- Post-infective scar/granuloma.
- Round pneumonia.
- Rheumatoid nodule (usually multiple).
- Infarct.

Multiple lung masses

- Multiple metastases.
- Vasculitis.
- Rheumatoid nodules.
- Multiple emboli.
- Multi focal infection.
- Progressive massive fibrosis (PMF).

Pleural effusion

- Large, unilateral.
  - Mesothelioma.
  - Metastatic pleural tumour.
  - Empyema.
- Small/moderate, unilateral:
  - Parapneumonic (associated with consolidation).
  - Empyema.
  - Malignancy (as above).
- Bilateral:
  - Heart failure.
  - Fluid overload.
  - Hypoalbuminaemia.

Cardiomegaly

- LV failure.
- Pericardial effusion.

Unilateral hyperradiancy

- Rotation of the patient.
- Pneumothorax.
- Chest wall abnormality:
  - Mastectomy.
  - Poland's syndrome.

Bilateral hyperradiancy

- Bilateral pneumothorax.
- Over expanded lungs:
  - Chronic obstructive pulmonary disease (COPD).
  - Asthma.

Upper zone fibrosis

- Sarcoid.
- Tuberculosis (TB).
- Post radiation.
- Pneumoconiosis.
- Extrinsic allergic alveolitis (EAA; chronic).
- Ankylosing spondylitis.

Small fibrotic lungs

- Idiopathic pulmonary fibrosis.
- Drug-induced fibrosis.
- Asbestosis.
- Connective tissue disease.

Kerley B lines

- Heart failure.
- Lymphangitis.
- Sarcoid.

Bilateral hilar enlargement

- Sarcoid.
- Pulmonary hypertension.
- Lymphoma.

Unilateral hilar enlargement

- Lung cancer.
- TB.
- Infection.

Respiratory presenting syndromes

Chest pain

This symptom is associated with a variety of disease processes, many of which are common and potentially life threatening. A possible myocardial infarction must be the first consideration in all adults with acute chest pain. Once this has been excluded, the list of differential diagnoses can be narrowed by accurate interpretation of history, examination, and investigations (Table 3.1).

Investigations

These will be guided by the presentation and likely diagnosis. In general, an electrocardiogram (ECG) is required to rule out cardiac ischaemia/infarction as well as a plain chest radiograph. A summary of available imaging tests relevant in the investigation of chest pain are briefly described in the 'Imaging' section. More detailed applications and findings will be discussed under each relevant condition.

Imaging

Plain chest radiograph

This may prove to be diagnostic. It may show signs of cardiac failure, pneumothorax, or collapse/consolidation. Mediastinal widening, shift, and the presence of free gas can all be detected.

Ultrasound

Ultrasound examination of the heart (echocardiography) can be used to detect aortic arch aneurysms, dissecting aneurysms, cardiomayopathy and pericardial effusion. Transoesophageal echocardiography (TOE) has been developed to overcome limitations of conventional echocardiography in trying to image through the anterior chest wall.

Ultrasound examination of the chest can be used to detect the presence of pleural fluid and to guide aspiration/drainage.

CT

Can be used to evaluate/diagnose dissecting thoracic aneurysms, pericardial effusions, and myocardial tumours. More advanced scanners allow non-invasive assessment of the coronary arteries. Recent NICE guidelines recommend unenhanced CT to assess coronary artery calcification in cases of atypical chest pain.

Respiratory causes of chest pain can be evaluated with CT, including CT pulmonary angiography (CTPA) for suspected cases of pulmonary embolism.

CT also allows evaluation of the pleural space and chest wall.

Nuclear medicine

Thallium (^{201}Tl) exercise test

Not used in the acute setting but can differentiate viable from non-viable myocardium and hence identify those patients who would benefit from coronary revascularization. Following injection with ^{201}Tl, imaging is performed immediately after exercise and then repeated 4 hours later.

Ventilation/perfusion imaging
Combined perfusion scanning with technetium-99m-labelled macroaggregates of human albumin and ventilation scanning with inhaled radioactive gas or aerosol to assess possible pulmonary embolus.

MRI
Little role in acute setting. Has some value in assessing pericardial effusions, hypertrophic cardiomyopathy, and congenital/valvular heart disease. MR angiography provides a non-invasive method of imaging vascular abnormalities such as aneurysm and dissection, but does not have the spatial resolution necessary to assess the coronary arteries.

Arteriography
Coronary angiography
This is a commonly performed examination during which contrast is initially injected into the left ventricle to evaluate function, and subsequently into the coronary arteries to demonstrate the extent of any stenoses or occlusion. Angioplasty and stenting can then be performed if indicated.

Pulmonary angiography
This is an invasive procedure which is now rarely performed since the advent of CTPA. It involves selective catheterization of the pulmonary artery (either through the jugular or femoral vein) and contrast injection to visualize the pulmonary circulation.

Table 3.1 Differential diagnosis

Cardiac	Pulmonary	Other
Myocardial ischaemia/infarction*	Pneumothorax*	Oesophageal rupture with mediastinitis*
Aortic dissection*	Pulmonary embolus*	Pancreatitis*
Pericarditis	Pneumonia	Oesophagitis
Myocarditis	Lung cancer	Cholecystitis
Mitral valve prolapse	Mesothelioma	Herpes zoster (shingles)
	Pleural effusion	Costochondritis (Tietze's disease)
		Vertebral collapse
		Trauma

* Potentially rapidly life threatening

Wheeze

Wheeze is the sound produced by the vibration of narrowed airways. Normally heard best in expiration, wheeze can be either polyphonic, with multiple different pitches and volumes, or monophonic with a single constant pitch.

Wheeze which can only be heard in inspiration is termed stridor and is indicative of an upper respiratory tract cause.

A localized or fixed wheeze is suspicious of tumour or foreign body within an airway.

Polyphonic wheeze

- Asthma.
- COPD.
- Cardiac failure.
- Anaphylaxis.
- Extrinsic allergic alveolitis (EAA).
- Chondromalacia.
- Pneumonia (less common).

Monophonic wheeze

- Bronchial carcinoma.
- Foreign body.

Stridor

- Anaphylaxis.
- Peritonsilar or retropharyngeal abscess.
- Epiglottitis/croup.
- Foreign body.
- Pharyngeal pouch.
- Thyroid goitre.
- Upper respiratory tract neoplasm.
- Vocal cord paralysis.
- Rarely congenital vascular abnormalities/rings in children.

Imaging

In acute life-threatening airway obstruction imaging is a distraction. The patient requires urgent clinical management. Once the patient is stabilized imaging may play a role.

Plain film

- Chest x-ray (CXR) can identify tumour, foreign bodies, cardiac failure, or infection.
- Background conditions such as COPD may be evident.
- In acute asthma the CXR may be normal or show only large volume lungs, but is useful to exclude pneumothorax or exacerbating conditions such as infection.
- A lateral cervical spine x-ray may identify radio-opaque foreign bodies or rarely a fluid level in a retropharyngeal abscess.

CT

- CT of neck and chest may reveal extrinsic airway compression by mass lesions, endoluminal lesions within the airways, or congenital abnormalities.
- Expiratory CT can demonstrate focal areas of air trapping in patients with small airways disease and collapse of the larger airways in those with bronchomalacia.

Ultrasound

Ultrasound is not routinely used to investigate wheeze. Neck masses such as nodes or goitre can be assessed.

Fluoroscopy /nuclear medicine/MRI

These are not routinely used. However a barium swallow will diagnose a pharyngeal pouch or identify extrinsic oesophageal compression which may indicate pathology such as vascular rings that are also causing airway compression.

Information for the radiologist

- Any history of background lung conditions.
- Has a foreign body been inhaled (some are not radio-opaque)?
- Location of the wheeze.
- Any history of smoking, cancer, or congenital abnormality.
- Respiratory function tests.
- Is there a seasonal picture or anything to suggest allergy?

Shortness of breath

A common problem with a wide range of causes. The key to narrowing the differential diagnosis lies in accurate history taking and examination.

Presentation

Presentation varies according to the cause. Associated symptoms should be elicited. The duration of illness is helpful to narrow the differential diagnosis:

- Sudden onset (over minutes):
  - Pneumothorax: pleuritic chest pain. May be a history of trauma.
  - Myocardial infarction: chest pain, sweating, clammy.
  - Pulmonary embolus: pleuritic chest pain, haemoptysis, syncope.
  - Inhaled foreign body: often in children, cyanosis, stridor.
  - Anaphylaxis: stridor, tongue/throat swelling, urticarial rash.
- Acute (onset over hours):
  - Asthma: expiratory wheeze, chest pain.
  - Pneumonia: fever, productive cough, coarse crepitations.
  - Pulmonary oedema: widespread inspiratory crepitations.
  - Cardiac tamponade: muffled heart sounds, raised jugular venous pressure (JVP), hypotension.
  - Metabolic acidosis: e.g. diabetic ketoacidosis. Check glucose, arterial blood gases (ABG).
  - Inappropriate hyperventilation.
- Chronic (onset over months):
  - Asthma.
  - COPD: history of smoking, wheeze and recurrent chest infections.
  - Interstitial lung disease: e.g. idiopathic pulmonary fibrosis.
  - Heart failure: worse on exertion, orthopnoea, peripheral oedema.
  - Pulmonary hypertension: chest pain, fatigue, right heart failure.
  - Lung cancer: weight loss, cough, haemoptysis, smoking history.
  - Anaemia: pallor. Check full blood count (FBC).

Adjuncts to clinical examination include ECG, ABG, routine blood tests, and pulse oximetry.

Imaging

Plain film

CXR is the initial imaging investigation. It may identify many of the acute causes, e.g. pneumothorax, pleural effusion, cardiac failure, pneumonia. Also useful to compare with old radiographs in cases of chronic dyspnoea.

CT

Occasionally required if the diagnosis cannot be made on plain film. Performed as high resolution CT (HRCT), CTPA, or normal contrast enhanced CT depending on the clinical question.

Nuclear medicine

V/Q scans are used to identify pulmonary emboli.

Ultrasound

May demonstrate pleural or pericardial effusions.

Information for the radiologist

- Presenting symptoms and duration of illness.
- Relevant past medical history, e.g. cardiac disease, smoking, allergy.
- Clinical differential diagnosis.

Cough

Cough is a common presenting complaint and there are a wide range of causes, of which upper respiratory tract infection is the most common.

Presentation

Presentation varies according to the cause. The nature of the cough should be explored:

- Duration: acute or chronic (see later in topic).
- Productivity: dry, sputum, blood.
- Timing: e.g. worse in early morning (asthma), following food (reflux).
- Environmental precipitants: e.g. drugs, pets, smoking, exercise.

Associated symptoms may include nasal discharge, fever, wheeze, dyspnoea, peripheral oedema, weight loss, or recurrent chest infections and provide important clues as to the underlying aetiology.

The duration of symptoms can be used to classify causes:

- Acute (<3 weeks):
  - Upper respiratory tract infection.
  - Lower respiratory tract infection and pneumonia.
  - Airway disease: e.g. asthma, COPD.
  - Heart failure.
  - Aspiration.
  - Extrinsic allergic alveolitis: e.g. pigeon fancier's lung.
  - Pulmonary embolus.
- Chronic (>3 weeks):
  - Post-nasal drip.
  - Airway disease: COPD, asthma, lung cancer, bronchiectasis.
  - Interstitial lung disease.
  - Extrinsic allergic alveolitis.
  - Heart failure.
  - Gastro-oesophageal reflux disease with recurrent aspiration.
  - Drugs: e.g. angiotensin converting enzyme (ACE) inhibitors.

Imaging

Plain film

Recommended if symptoms last 3 weeks or more. A good screening tool if there is concern for a pulmonary or cardiac cause.

CT

Persistent cough is sometimes investigated with CT, particularly if there is concern for malignancy, bronchiectasis, or interstitial lung disease.

Ultrasound

Echocardiography is a reliable method of assessing cardiac function.

Fluoroscopy

Contrast swallow examinations can demonstrate gastro-oesophageal reflux and aspiration.

Information for the radiologist
- Nature of cough and associated symptoms.
- Relevant environmental history e.g. pets, occupational history, smoking.

Haemoptysis

Haemoptysis is the coughing up of blood from the lungs or tracheobronchial tree (Table 3.2). Massive haemoptysis refers to the coughing up of >200ml of blood in 24 hours.

Imaging

The cause of haemoptysis may be obvious from the history and investigations should be performed according to the likely diagnosis.

Plain film

This should be performed in all patients presenting with haemoptysis. It may reveal a mass lesion, mediastinal lymphadenopathy, bronchiectasis, cavitation, consolidation, or pulmonary oedema.

Ultrasound

Ultrasound examination of the heart (echocardiography) can be used to detect cardiac causes of haemoptysis including anatomical abnormalities, valvular disease, and ventricular dysfunction.

CT

CT of the chest may identify parenchymal or endobronchial lesions, or further characterize abnormalities seen on plain chest radiograph.

HRCT is performed where generalized lung disease is suspected (e.g. bronchiectasis). Traditional intermittent HRCT uses widely spaced, thin sections and is therefore unsuitable for the assessment of lung cancer or other localized lung diseases. Similarly, IV contrast agents are not routinely administered making the technique unsuitable for assessment of soft tissues and blood vessels.

CTPA is commonly performed for suspected pulmonary embolism. In this test, iodinated contrast is administered intravenously to opacify the pulmonary arterial tree. Any filling defects indicate the presence of a pulmonary embolus.

In cases of massive haemoptysis contrast enhanced CT can be useful in identifying enlarged bronchial arteries which may be suitable for embolization.

Nuclear medicine

V/Q imaging should be considered for patients with suspected pulmonary embolism who have a normal chest radiograph and no known history of respiratory disease. Combined perfusion scanning with technetium-99m-labelled macroaggregates of human albumin and ventilation scanning with inhaled radioactive gas or aerosol typically produces a perfusion defect and not a ventilation defect in pulmonary embolus.

MRI

The lungs are not well visualized with MR and its use in the assessment of respiratory causes of haemoptysis is limited.

Angiography
Pulmonary angiography can identify the bleeding source in 90% of patients with massive haemoptysis and can be combined with embolization of the bleeding vessel.

Other
Fibreoptic bronchoscopy may be used in cases of suspected malignancy. It is diagnostic for central endobronchial lesions and allows direct visualization of the bleeding site. In cases of more peripheral bleeding the bronchoscopist may be able to identify the affected lobe, which is useful information for a vascular radiologist considering embolization. It also permits tissue biopsy, bronchial lavage, or brushings for pathological diagnosis.

Table 3.2 Differential diagnosis

Pulmonary	Cardiac	Systemic vasculitis
Bronchiectasis	Pulmonary embolus	Systemic lupus erythematosus (SLE)
Bronchogenic carcinoma	Left ventricular failure	Wegener's granulomatosis
Infection	Mitral stenosis	Goodpasture's syndrome
TB	Pulmonary hypertension	
Pneumonia	Aortic aneurysm (aorto-bronchial fistula)	
Lung abscess		
Aspergilloma		
Trauma		
AV malformation		

Hypoxia

Hypoxia is defined as reduced oxygen supply to tissues despite adequate blood supply. Possible causes are listed:

1. Reduced oxygen carrying capacity

- Anaemia.
- Carbon monoxide poisoning.
- Haemoglobinopathies (e.g. sickle cell, thalassaemia).

2. Reduced blood supply to lungs

- Pulmonary embolism (thrombus, fat, amniotic).
- Right-sided heart failure.
- Pulmonary hypertension.
- Pulmonary valve stenosis.
- Congenital heart disease.

3. Reduced diffusion of oxygen across the alveolar membrane

- Upper airway obstruction (e.g. foreign body).
- Lower airway pathology (e.g. asthma/COPD/tumour).
- Material within alveoli:
  - Inflammatory cells (infection/hypersensitivity).
  - Pulmonary haemorrhage.
  - Pulmonary oedema.
  - Tumour.
- Interstitial lung disease/fibrosis.
- Bronchiectasis/cystic fibrosis.
- Collapse of lung due to pneumothorax or pleural effusion.
- Neuromuscular disorders (e.g. Guillain–Barré syndrome).

Imaging

Plain film

- A CXR is likely to be the first form of imaging used to investigate the hypoxic patient. It is most useful for the 3rd category of causes listed earlier.
- Cardiac and mediastinal abnormalities may suggest a cause from the 2nd category.
- Remember CXR signs may lag behind the clinical findings.

CT

- Standard CT **thorax ± contrast** provides detailed 3D information.
- CTPA is the investigation of choice for detecting pulmonary emboli.
- HRCT acquires 1mm slices to assess the structures of the small airways and interstitium. Used in the diagnosis of interstitial lung disease and atypical infection.
- Cardiac CT assesses cardiac structure and function; however is usually performed after an echocardiogram.

Ultrasound
- Ultrasound can confirm pleural effusions or pneumothorax prior to guided intervention.
- Echocardiography evaluates cardiac structure and function.

Nuclear medicine
V/Q scanning can be used to investigate pulmonary embolism if immediately available but should only be used in those patients with a normal CXR and no previous cardiorespiratory disease.

MRI
Cardiac MRI assesses structure and function of the heart but is usually a second-line examination.

Information for the radiologist
- Relevant history including previous respiratory disease, smoking, immunosuppression, malignancy, or previous surgery.
- A differential diagnosis is vital to choose the most appropriate investigation.

Respiratory conditions

Lung abscess

A lung abscess is a well-defined collection of pus, usually with a discrete wall and surrounded by inflamed lung tissue. They usually develop as a complication of bacterial pneumonia and may be solitary or multiple.

Clinical presentation

The clinical course is often insidious, with fever, lethargy, and night sweats. Breathlessness and productive cough with haemoptysis may be present.

- If due to aspiration, abscesses often involve the posterior segments of the upper lobes and the apical segments of the lower lobes, as these areas are gravity dependent when the patient is supine.
- Systemic bacteraemia or tricuspid valve endocarditis can cause multiple septic emboli throughout the lungs leading to abscess formation.
- Secondary abscess formation can occur within pre-existing cavities (bullae or lung cysts), or distal to an obstructed bronchus, e.g. secondary to a carcinoma or inhaled foreign body.

Imaging

Plain film

Chest radiographs may not be diagnostic in the early stages of abscess formation, often showing a non-specific area of consolidation, before progressing to the classical appearance of a well-defined mass with an air-fluid level (Fig. 4.1). Remember, the air-fluid level will only be present on upright films.

Ultrasound

Limited role in imaging the abscess itself, but echo is useful if septic emboli from endocarditis considered.

CT

- Identifies cavitation within an area of consolidation.
- Delineates the position of the abscess with respect to bronchial anatomy and the chest wall (Fig. 4.2).
- Useful for differentiating between intrapulmonary abscess and loculated empyema.
- Furthermore, CT is invaluable for accurate placement of drainage catheters, if required.

Information for the radiologist

- Is the patient septic?
- Is the patient at risk of aspiration or is there a history such as an alcoholism, immunosuppression, epilepsy, or dysphagia?
- Before considering percutaneous drainage appropriate broad-spectrum antibiotics should usually have been given a suitable trial first.
- If drainage is being requested lung function and INR will be required.

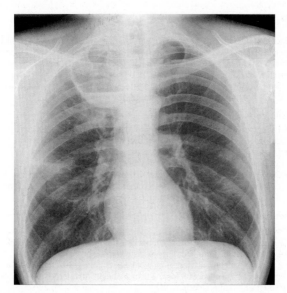

Fig. 4.1 CXR of a 35-year-old man with fever and purulent cough showing a thin-walled abscess in the right lung apex containing an air fluid level.

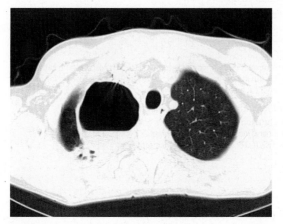

Fig. 4.2 CT of same patient as Fig. 4.1 confirming the position and nature of the abscess in the right upper lobe with small amount of surrounding consolidation. Note the thin, smooth wall and air fluid level. (Patient grew *Staph. aureus* from blood cultures and abscess resolved with antibiotic treatment.)

Pneumonia

Bacterial pneumonias are categorized by their infectious agents, which include *Streptococcus pneumoniae* (the most common cause of bacterial pneumonias), *Haemophilus influenzae*, *Klebsiella*, *Staphylococcus*, *Legionella* species, and Gram-negative organisms.

Susceptibility to pneumonias increase with very young or old age, COPD, alcoholism, and immunocompromise.

Clinical presentation

- Patients may present with cough productive of sputum (green or rust coloured), rigors, malaise, myalgia, dyspnoea, or pleuritic chest pain.
- *Legionella* pneumonia is associated with GI symptoms including anorexia, nausea, vomiting, and diarrhoea.
- Signs are legion, and include fever, wheeze, tachypnoea, tachycardia, dullness on percussion, decreased breath sounds, rhonchi and rales on auscultation, and a pleural friction rub.

Imaging

Plain film (Fig. 4.3)

CXR is the initial investigation in most cases and important in follow-up.
- Lobar consolidation (ill defined opacity with air bronchograms).
- Cavitating pneumonia and bulging of fissures is suggestive of *Klebsiella*, (which has a predilection for the upper lobes), *Staphylococcus aureus* or TB (see 📖 Tuberculosis, p. 86).
- Pleural effusion.
- Abscess.
- Lobar collapse.

Ultrasound

No role in uncomplicated pneumonia but useful to identify and localize secondary effusions/empyema.

CT

- Not needed in uncomplicated cases which resolve on treatment.
- Useful in non-resolving infection to look for an obstructing lesion or atypical features such as cavitation.

Information for the radiologist

- Duration of symptoms.
- Bronchoscopy results if relevant.
- Risk factors including immunosuppression.

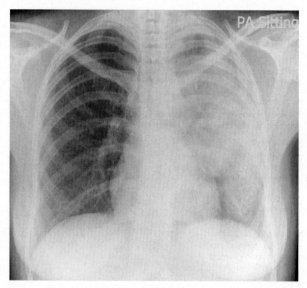

Fig. 4.3 CXR showing extensive consolidation throughout the left lung, due to proven streptococcal pneumonia.

Emphysema/COPD

Emphysema is defined as irreversible dilatation of the airways distal to the terminal bronchiole, accompanied by the destruction of alveolar walls and without obvious fibrosis.

Frequently occurs in association with bronchitis and these entities are referred to with the collective term chronic obstructive pulmonary disease (COPD).

Clinical presentation

Patients typically present in their 5th/6th decade with breathlessness and productive cough. Smoking is a common factor.

Clinical signs
- Hyperinflation, i.e. 'barrel chest'.
- Wheezing.
- Hyperresonance on percussion.

Imaging

Plain film (Figs. 4.4 and 4.5)
- Increased lung volumes (increased AP diameter on lateral).
- Flattened diaphragms.
- Hyperlucency of lungs.
- Reduction in number and calibre of vascular shadows.
- Bullae (air spaces that measure >1cm in diameter).

CT

Emphysema is usually an incidental finding as CT is not used in the routine care of patients with COPD.

CT is indicated in those patients who are undergoing evaluation for surgical intervention, i.e. bullectomy or lung volume reduction surgery.

Typical findings include:
- Extensive areas of low attenuation without definable walls.
- Thin walled avascular areas (bullae).
- Paucity of vascular markings in affected areas.
- Upper lobe predominance in centrilobular and paraseptal emphysema.
- Lower lobe predominance in panacinar emphysema (feature of alpha-1 antitrypsin deficiency).

Nuclear medicine
V/Q scanning is performed to assess relative lung function and distribution of disease prior to lung volume reduction surgery.

Information for the radiologist
- Smoking history.
- Duration of symptoms.
- Respiratory function tests.

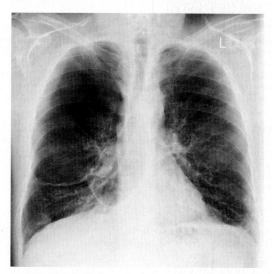

Fig. 4.4 PA CXR showing bullous emphysema throughout most of the right upper lobe. Note the absence of lung markings in the right upper and mid zones and the depression of the horizontal fissure.

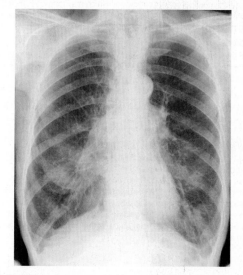

Fig. 4.5 PA CXR showing overexpanded lungs and flattening of the hemidiaphragms typical of COPD.

Pulmonary embolus

A pulmonary embolism (PE) is a blockage of the pulmonary artery, or its branches. This may be acute, most commonly a clot from a DVT, or chronic, due to longstanding thromboembolic disease.

Other, less common causes include fat, tumour, air, and amniotic fluid emboli.

The ideal imaging protocols for diagnosing PE remain a subject of debate amongst radiologists.

Clinical presentation

Classically, patients present with pleuritic chest pain, breathlessness, a swollen leg, and ECG changes but PE may present with symptoms ranging from vague breathlessness to cardiac arrest.

Risk factors include:
- Recent immobilization.
- Recent surgery.
- Previous PE/DVT.
- Smoking.
- Pregnancy/oral contraceptive pill.
- Thrombophilic disorders including malignancy.

Imaging features

Plain film
- Non-specific and up to 40% of patients with acute PE have a normal CXR.
- Will quickly exclude other conditions which may mimic PE, including pneumothorax, pneumonia and aortic dissection, and is important in deciding which imaging modality will subsequently be used.

Ultrasound
As the treatment for above-knee DVT and PE is the same, ultrasound scanning and demonstration of a DVT mitigates the need for further investigation.

Echocardiography
- Assessment of right heart strain in acute PE (and may visualize large clot in central pulmonary arteries).
- Right ventricular hypertrophy in chronic embolic disease.

CTPA (Fig. 4.6)
- Emboli are seen as intraluminal filling defects within the contrast enhanced pulmonary arteries.
- When clot is seen the PPV is high, but these studies can be difficult to interpret, particularly in the context of respiratory motion artefact and poorly opacified pulmonary vessels.
- CTPA has the advantage of providing additional information not possible with perfusion scanning, such as the presence of right heart strain and infarcted lung.

Ventilation/perfusion scanning (Fig. 4.7)
- Radioisotope assessment of ventilation (using inhaled agents such as Xe-133, Tc-99m aerosol) and lung perfusion (using a venous injection of Tc-99m macroaggregated albumin) is the traditional method of PE diagnosis and remains a commonly used test in many departments.
- A high probability scan is very accurate in confirming the presence of PE, whilst a normal study excludes significant PE.
- However, a significant proportion of the studies are indeterminate and further imaging is needed.
- The chances of an indeterminate scan are much higher in those with an abnormal CXR, hence these patients are normally sent straight to CT.

MRI
- MRI of the pulmonary vasculature is possible; however, spatial and contrast resolution is inferior to CTPA, and MR in acute PE is rarely used.
- In chronic embolic disease MRA combined with assessment of right ventricular function is commonly used in pre-treatment work-up.

Pulmonary angiography
Conventional pulmonary angiography is still nominally the gold standard for the diagnosis of PE. However, it is an interventional procedure (overall complication rate is 2–5%) and is now rarely performed outside of specialist centres.

Information for the radiologist
- Pretest probability (including D-dimer).
- Does the patient have asthma or chronic lung disease?

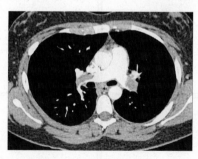

Fig. 4.6 Axial image from CTPA reveals filling defects in both main pulmonary arteries in keeping with pulmonary emboli.

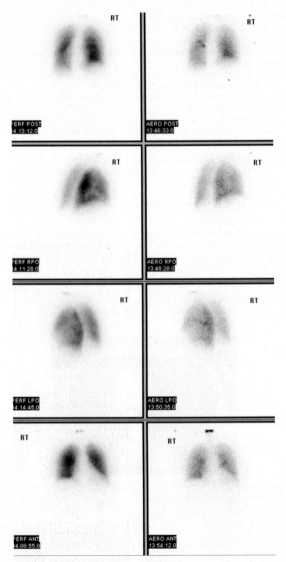

Fig. 4.7 Image from V/Q scan from a different patient than Fig. 4.6 demonstrating the normal appearance bilaterally. This pattern virtually excludes PE.

Left ventricular failure

Failure of the left ventricle to pump adequately, either as a consequence of systolic dysfunction (a reduction of myocardial contractility), diastolic dysfunction (an abnormality of distensibility), or a combination of the two.

Clinical presentation

Worsening breathlessness, orthopnoea, basal crepitations, wheeze and respiratory failure may all indicate left ventricular failure (LVF).

Onset may be acute or insidious. In patients with limited cardiac reserve, a separate episode such as a chest infection may precipitate acute LVF.

LVF may develop following acute MI due to the loss of functioning myocardium, arrhythmias, papillary muscle rupture, ventricular septal defect (VSD), or transmural infarct resulting in haemopericardium.

Imaging

Plain film

The radiographic changes centre on cardiomegaly (cardiothoracic ratio >55%) and pulmonary oedema.

As the pulmonary capillary wedge pressure (PCWP) rises, cephalization of the pulmonary vasculature (upper lobar venous diversion) develops.

Interstitial oedema is the next sign, as evidenced by peribronchial cuffing, loss of clarity to vessels, fluid in the fissures, and development of interstitial lines:

- Kerley A lines radiate out from the hila.
- Kerley B lines: short horizontal lines in the lung peripheries (Fig. 4.8).

Further rises in PCWP lead to the development of alveolar pulmonary oedema, seen as bilateral air-space shadowing and pleural effusions.

In this phase, it may be radiologically impossible to differentiate heart failure from severe infection.

Echocardiogram

Features of LVF include poor ejection fraction (EF), poor wall motion and contractility, and enlarged left ventricular chamber volumes.

Nuclear medicine

Very limited role in the imaging in acute LVF.

MRI

- Limited role in the acute setting.
- MRI is the most accurate modality for assessing LV function as well as myocardial reserve. It is also useful in assessing cardiomyopathy and the underlying cause.

CT

Limited role in the acute setting but can demonstrate causes such as acute VSD following infarction.

Information for the radiologist
- Any underlying cardiac condition which may be responsible for acute LVF should be mentioned.
- One common question is differentiation between LVF and chest infection which can be difficult purely on plain films.
- Clinical story and laboratory results will be needed to complete the picture.

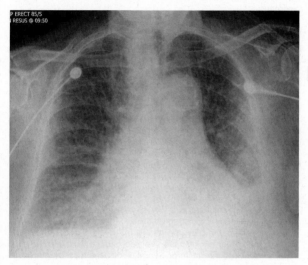

Fig. 4.8 PA CXR revealing cardiomegaly, upper lobe venous distension, Kerley B lines, and thickened interstitial markings in keeping with interstitial oedema secondary to heart failure. Note also the left pleural effusion.

Pneumothorax

A pneumothorax occurs when air enters the pleural cavity, separating the visceral from the parietal pleura, with subsequent collapse of the underlying lung. The air can be free within the pleural cavity, loculated, or under tension, causing haemodynamic compromise and instability.

Spontaneous pneumothoraces are more common in asthmatics, patients with emphysema, cystic fibrosis, and TB. There is also a predisposition to spontaneous pneumothorax in tall thin males (and those with Marfan's syndrome).

Traumatic pneumothorax is often the result of chest wall compression or penetrating injury with lung laceration.

Remember iatrogenic causes, such as insertion of central venous lines, lung biopsies, radiotherapy, and positive pressure ventilation.

Clinical presentation

Pneumothorax can present with sudden onset of chest pain and breathlessness, or, in the case of tension pneumothorax, with cardiovascular compromise and collapse.

It is an important diagnosis to exclude in the context of trauma, where small pneumothoraces may go undetected on the supine CXR, resulting in rapid decompression should positive pressure ventilation be needed.

In cases of tension pneumothorax the patient may be tachycardic, hypotensive, and tachypnoeic.

Imaging features

Plain film (Figs. 4.9 and 4.10)

The visceral pleura is seen as a thin curvilinear line which parallels the chest wall (a skin fold is usually much thicker).

The air within the chest cavity will make the hemithorax appear 'blacker', and no lung markings are visible beyond the line of pleura.

The presence of rib fractures, subcutaneous emphysema, and bullae should provoke a thorough search for a pneumothorax.

Signs of a tension pneumothorax on CXR include:
- Unilateral hyperlucency.
- Deviated trachea and mediastinum away from the abnormal side.
- Depression of the ipsilateral hemidiaphragm.

The immediate response is needle decompression.

Remember—when the patient is supine a pneumothorax is more difficult to detect, as the air collects superiorly, overlying the lungs, and the pleural edge is often not visible. The heart borders and diaphragms become unusually well defined. The affected lung base becomes lucent (black) which progresses to the deep sulcus sign, where the costophrenic angle is depressed, as pressure increases.

Ultrasound

Ultrasound can be used to diagnose pneumothorax (in specialist hands!) However, it is rarely used in the acute setting.

CT

CT is the gold standard test for detecting and localizing pneumothorax, and may be necessary to guide percutaneous drainage.

In addition, CT can help clarify the presence of bullae, which may simulate pneumothorax on the plain film.

Information for the radiologist

- Any history of trauma.
- Previous history of pneumothorax.
- Recent iatrogenic procedure.

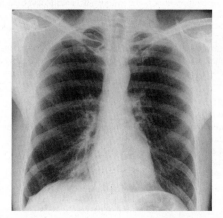

Fig. 4.9 CXR of patient with sudden onset of chest pain and dyspnoea, showing a pleural edge at the right apex with absent lung markings lateral to it, indicating a pneumothorax. Note that the mediastinum remains central and the diaphragms are normally positioned.

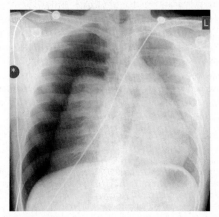

Fig. 4.10 CXR of a tension pneumothorax on the right. The collapsed lung is opacified, the mediastinum is shifted away from the affected side and the ipsilateral diaphragm is depressed. This needs urgent decompression.

Wegener's granulomatosis

Disease of unknown aetiology causing granulomatous inflammation of small- and medium-sized blood vessels in the respiratory tract, kidneys, and other organs.

Clinical presentation

- Upper respiratory tract symptoms: rhinitis, sinusitis and otitis media.
- Pulmonary involvement is very common (up to 90%) and may cause dyspnoea, cough, haemoptysis, chest pain, or stridor due to airway stenosis.
- Progressive renal failure secondary to necrotizing glomerulonephritis.
- Arthralgia and myalgia.
- Epistaxis.
- Scleritis.

Imaging

Plain film (Figs. 4.11 and 4.12)

- Patchy infiltrates and consolidation due to pulmonary haemorrhage.
- Cavitating nodules.
- Pleural effusion.
- Atelectasis.
- Pneumothorax (uncommon).

Nodules and consolidation may resolve without a trace over a period of months leaving a normal radiograph.

CT

- Tracheal/bronchial stenosis (can be life threatening).
- Nodules which frequently cavitate. These may be surrounded by a 'halo' of ground glass opacification due to haemorrhage.
- Peripheral pulmonary infarcts.

CT of the sinuses will show any nasal involvement.

Ultrasound

Renal ultrasound may show small kidneys of increased echogenicity, and guide biopsy.

Nuclear medicine

Active areas of disease will show increased uptake on gallium scans.

MRI

Brain/spinal imaging may show neuritis.

Information for the radiologist

- Presenting symptoms.
- Renal function.
- Vasculitic screen: c-ANCA (centrally accentuated antineutrophil cytoplasmic antibody test): usually but not always positive.
- Past medical history (e.g. malignancy, PE, rheumatoid disease, immunosuppression) will help to guide differential diagnosis.
- Consideration of lung/renal biopsy? (Would need current blood tests including coagulation screen.)

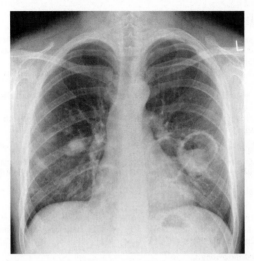

Fig. 4.11 CXR of a young man revealing several cavitating mass lesions in both lungs. The patient presented with vasculitic rash, haematuria, and dyspnoea.

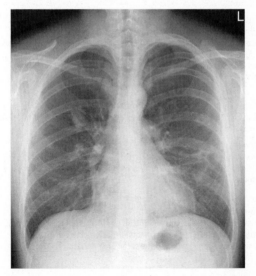

Fig. 4.12 CXR of the same patient as Fig. 4.11 several months later following immunosuppressive treatment. The lesions have all regressed, leaving residual scar tissue and atelectasis.

Pulmonary hypertension

Defined as sustained systolic pulmonary artery pressure of >25mmHg at rest or >30mmHg during exercise with increased pulmonary vascular resistance.

May be primary (idiopathic) or secondary to cardiac, pulmonary or hepatic disease. Causes include:
- Increased pulmonary blood flow secondary to congenital heart disease or high-output cardiac states.
- Increased pulmonary vascular resistance, e.g. PE, connective tissue diseases, pulmonary fibrosis, or pulmonary venous hypertension.

Clinical presentation

Chest pain, dyspnoea, haemoptysis, fatigue, or syncope. There may be signs of right heart failure (raised JVP, hepatomegaly, ascites, oedema).

Imaging

Plain film (Fig. 4.13)

CXR may reveal cardiomegaly and enlarged central pulmonary arteries with peripheral pruning. There may be signs of underlying pulmonary parenchymal disease, e.g. COPD.

Echocardiography

Demonstrates right ventricular hypertrophy and tricuspid regurgitation and is a non-invasive method of estimating pulmonary arterial pressure.

CT

May reveal:
- Right atrial and ventricular hypertrophy.
- Enlarged central pulmonary arteries, occasionally with calcification.
- Pruning of peripheral arteries.
- Pulmonary emboli.
- Pulmonary parenchymal disease.

MRI

Evaluates cardiac chambers, wall motion, stroke volume, and right ventricular EF (often reduced). Can also be used to depict pulmonary vasculature and assess shunts.

Pulmonary angiography

Allows accurate measurement of arterial pressures. Right heart catheterization can be performed to assess cardiac function and pulmonary flow dynamics.

Information for the radiologist

- Presenting symptoms.
- Relevant past medical history including risk factors for pulmonary hypertension, e.g. congenital heart disease, sickle cell anaemia.
- Clinical question, e.g. ?PE. ?Interstitial lung disease.

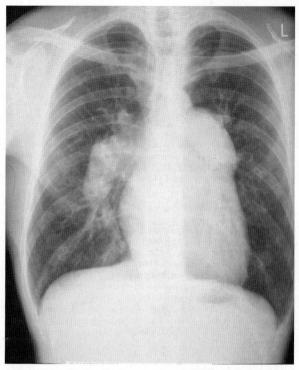

Fig. 4.13 CXR of a 54-year-old man with severe breathlessness reveals marked enlargement of the pulmonary trunk and main pulmonary arteries with relative oligaemia in the lungs themselves, in keeping with primary pulmonary hypertension.

Solitary pulmonary nodule

A single spherical lesion of 3cm or less in diameter, completely surrounded by lung without any associated atelectasis or lymphadenopathy.

Clinical presentation

Often an incidental finding on chest radiograph or CT. The main concern is usually to exclude malignancy. Discussion in multidisciplinary meetings is often required to define an appropriate management strategy.

Imaging

Plain film

CXR often identifies the solitary pulmonary nodule (SPN) initially. Dual-energy radiography can help determine if the nodule is calcified and does indeed lie within the lung. CXR may be able to characterize nodules but frequently CT is required (Figs. 4.14 and 4.15).

CT

More sensitive than plain film for detection of SPNs. May be used for characterization, to guide biopsy, or to monitor indeterminate nodules. To infer benignity, a nodule must be stable in volume for a period of at least 2 years. Certain features can help in characterization:

- Calcification: most patterns of calcification are associated with benign conditions such as hamartomas and TB. However, eccentric calcification is associated with malignancy.
- Density: e.g. fat indicates hamartoma or lipoma.
- Margins: speculated or smooth.
- Cavitation and wall thickness: thick-walled cavities suggest malignancy.
- Enhancement pattern: minimal enhancement suggests benignity.
- Size: unreliable but larger nodules are generally more likely to be malignant.

Nuclear medicine

Increased uptake on PET suggests malignancy though infection and inflammation can cause false positive results. PET lacks sensitivity for bronchoalveolar cell carcinoma and carcinoid, or if the nodule is <1cm in size.

MRI

With the advent of rapid acquisition sequences, MRI may have a role in the future.

Information for the radiologist

- Smoking history.
- Previous malignancy.
- Family history of lung cancer.
- Any previous imaging.
- Risk factors for TB, histoplasmosis.
- Current symptoms/signs of infection.
- Management plan if SPN already known.

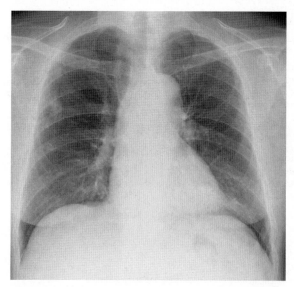

Fig. 4.14 CXR of a 60-year-old woman reveals a well-defined nodule in the right mid zone. There are no specific features to suggest a cause, and further investigation is required.

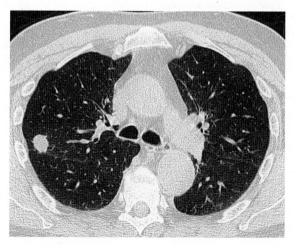

Fig. 4.15 CT of the same patient as Fig. 4.14 demonstrates the nodule lies in the right upper lobe, is solid, and has an irregular margin. CT biopsy revealed an adenocarcinoma and the patient underwent upper lobectomy.

Lung cancer

Lung cancer is the leading cause of cancer-related deaths in men and women worldwide and strongly associated with cigarette smoking.

Clinical presentation

Symptoms and signs are often non-specific, leading to a delay in diagnosis. Common symptoms include persistent cough, weight loss, haemoptysis, and chest pain.

Signs to look for include cachexia, finger clubbing, cervical/supraclavicular lymphadenopathy, reduced lung expansion, reduced breath sounds, or crepitations on auscultation.

Imaging

Plain film (Fig. 4.16)

Usually the initial imaging investigation. Look for:
- Signs of a mass.
- Mediastinal widening.
- Focal consolidation.
- Pleural effusion.
- Volume loss.
- Bone destruction.

CT (Fig. 4.17)

- Usual method of characterizing and staging disease.
- Important role in determining appropriate treatment pathways and prognosis.
- Much research currently ongoing into the feasibility of CT screening of at-risk individuals for early-stage lung cancer.
- Often used to obtain image-guided tissue biopsy.

Nuclear medicine

PET-CT has rapidly become a mainstay in the staging of potentially treatable disease and has been shown to detect significant numbers of metastases not seen with standard CT.

More accurate also in assessing mediastinal involvement than CT alone.

MRI

Used mostly as a problem solver in cases of spinal metastases, invasion of the chest apex by Pancoast tumours, and the characterization of adrenal masses.

Ultrasound

- Used for assessment and biopsy of neck nodes or liver metastases.
- Endoscopic/endobronchial ultrasound involves a small ultrasound probe on an endoscope for characterization and sampling of mediastinal nodes.

Information for the radiologist

Smoking history.

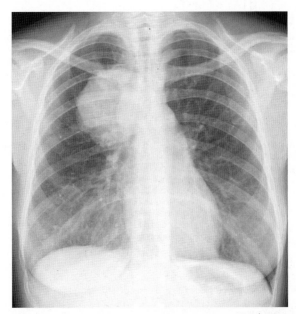

Fig. 4.16 CXR revealing a large right upper zone mass with widening of the right paratracheal stripe in a 55-year-old smoker.

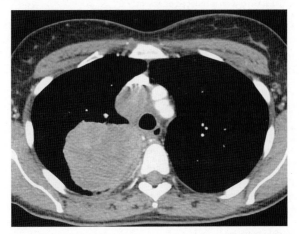

Fig. 4.17 CT of the same patients as Fig. 4.16 confirming the presence of a large lung cancer in the posterior segment of the right upper lobe and pathologically enlarged right paratracheal lymph nodes.

Lobar collapse

Atelectasis and collapse are interchangeable terms meaning diminished lung volume and deaeration.

The most common cause of lobar collapse is bronchial obstruction which may be due to:
- Mucus plugging.
- Inhaled foreign body.
- Endobronchial tumours.
- Extrinsic compression of the bronchus by tumour, lymphadenopathy, or aneurysm.

Atelectasis does not have to affect an entire lobe—smaller areas of lung may be affected by:
- Relaxation/passive atelectasis: due to space-occupying effects of pneumothorax, pleural effusion, or mass.
- Cicatrization atelectasis: volume loss due to fibrotic lung disease.
- Underexpansion of lung due to many causes including pain, chest wall abnormalities, diaphragmatic weakness.
- Adhesive atelectasis: complex and due to insufficient production of surfactant and is seen in respiratory distress syndrome (RDS) of the newborn.

Clinical presentation
Patients may present with:
- Dyspnoea: can be sudden if rapid onset of lobar collapse.
- Cyanosis.
- Chest pain.

Look for:
- Chest expansion is reduced or absent.
- The trachea and the heart are deviated toward the affected side.
- Dullness to percussion over the involved area.
- Reduced/absent breath sounds.

Imaging
Plain film
General signs of collapse:
- Displacement of fissures and opacification of the collapsed lobe.
- Displacement of the hilum (the left hilum is usually at least 1cm higher than right on a normal CXR).
- Mediastinal shift toward the collapse.
- Loss of volume.
- Compensatory hyperlucency of the remaining lobes.

For specific examples see Figs. 4.18–4.27.

CT
- This shows the same basic signs as on plain radiograph but to greater effect.
- Important role in detecting underlying lung tumours or other causes of bronchial obstruction.

Nuclear medicine
PET-CT is useful in detecting further sites of disease if malignancy has been confirmed.

Information for the radiologist
- Smoking history.
- Duration of symptoms.
- Suspicion of inhaled foreign body.
- Presence of haemoptysis.

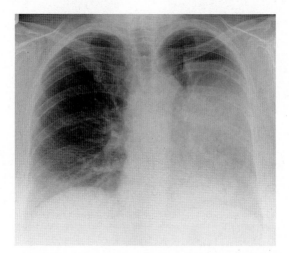

Fig. 4.18 Left upper lobe (LUL) collapse. PA CXR of LUL collapse, showing 'veil like' opacification of the left chest, obliteration of the heart border, elevation of the hilum, and preservation of the arch and descending thoracic aorta.

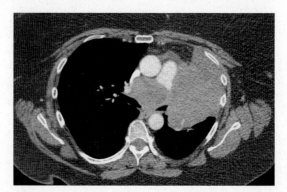

Fig. 4.19 CT scan of a different patient to Fig. 4.18 revealing LUL collapse due to a large tumour surrounding the hilar structures and invading the mediastinum. Note how the lobe collapses forwards to lie against the heart, while the lower lobe continues to outline the posterior structures such as the aorta.

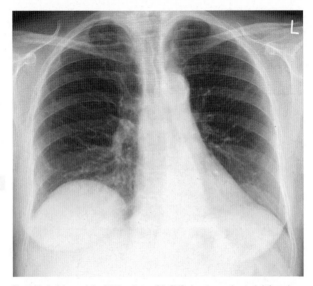

Fig. 4.20 Left lower lobe (LLL) collapse. PA CXR showing mediastinal shift to the left, depression of the left hilum and increased density behind the heart ('sail sign') due to LLL collapse.

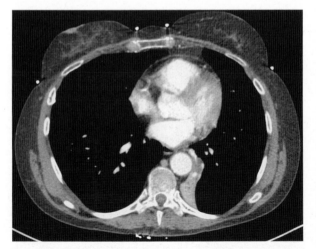

Fig. 4.21 Axial CT of patient with LLL collapse due to a low density mass at the hilum. Note how the lobe collapses medially, to lie against the spine.

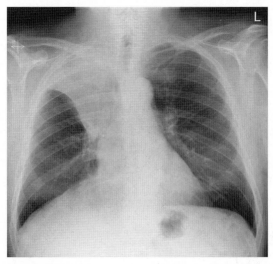

Fig. 4.22 Right upper lobe (RUL) collapse. PA CXR of patient with persistent cough, showing RUL collapse. The opacity in the right upper chest has a clearly defined, curved inferior border, consisting of the elevated horizontal fissure and the inferior border of a right hilar mass (the 'Golden S' sign). Note also mediastinal shift to the right and volume loss in the right chest.

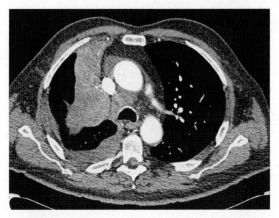

Fig. 4.23 Axial CT of the same patient as Fig. 4.22. The RUL has collapsed forwards to lie in the anterior chest. Note also enlarged right paratracheal nodes, pleural effusion, and trace of fluid in the pericardium around the ascending aorta.

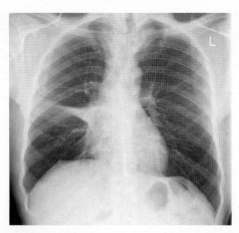

Fig. 4.24 Right middle lobe collapse. PA CXR revealing a well defined soft tissue density extending from the right hilum, associated with loss of clarity to the right heart border and minimal signs of volume loss.

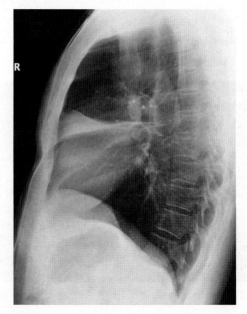

Fig. 4.25 Right lateral CXR of the same patient as Fig. 4.24, demonstrating the horizontal and oblique fissures drawn together as the middle lobe collapses between them.

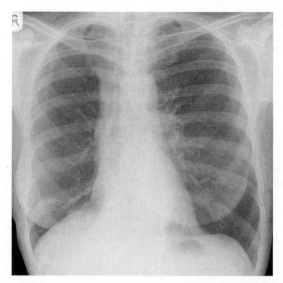

Fig. 4.26 Right lower lobe (RLL) collapse. PA CXR of patient with RLL collapse. Note volume loss to the right hemi thorax, depression of the right hilum, and the increased density of the collapsed lobe.

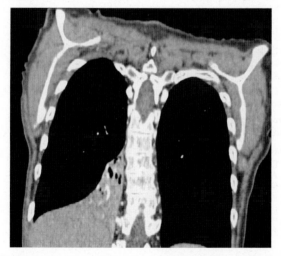

Fig. 4.27 Coronal reformat of CT scan showing collapse of the RLL. Appearances are similar to those on the left with the collapsed lobe lying posteriorly and medially against the spine.

Bronchiectasis

Irreversible dilatation of those bronchi which contain cartilage in their walls, leading to inflammation in the lung and impaired clearance of secretions. Causes include infections (particularly in childhood), cystic fibrosis, immunodeficiency, chronic aspiration, ciliary dysfunction, and proximal airway obstruction (e.g. by tumour or foreign body).

Clinical presentation

Chronic cough and sputum production, dyspnoea, haemoptysis, and recurrent chest infections. On examination there may be clubbing, weight loss, wheeze, and coarse crepitations in the lungs. Pulmonary function tests are normal or show an obstructive pattern.

Imaging

Plain film (Fig. 4.28)

Chest radiographs are the initial investigation but are often normal. 'Tubular' or 'cylindrical' bronchiectasis causes a 'tram-track' appearance of parallel lines caused by thick-walled dilated bronchi. Cystic structures with air-fluid levels may be seen in cystic bronchiectasis. Infection can cause alveolar consolidation.

CT (Fig. 4.29)

HRCT is the most sensitive test, demonstrating both the location and extent of disease. Findings include:
- Dilated bronchi with peribronchial thickening and mucus retention.
- Bronchi which do not taper peripherally, are larger in diameter than the accompanying pulmonary artery branch (signet-ring sign), and which reach the lung peripheries.
- Bronchoceles (bronchi filled with fluid).
- Cystic changes with air fluid levels.
- Crowding of vessels caused by volume loss.
- Compensatory emphysematous changes in non-affected areas.
- Fibrosis and honeycombing in more severe disease.
- Expiratory scans reveal areas of air trapping.

CT may also provide clues as to the cause of bronchiectasis, e.g. foreign bodies and bronchial tumours.

Bronchography

Now very rarely used.

Information for the radiologist

- Duration of symptoms.
- Any underlying pulmonary disease (e.g. tumour, cystic fibrosis, Kartagener's syndrome).
- Previous chest infections, particularly childhood infections.
- Immunodeficiency.
- Previous radiotherapy.

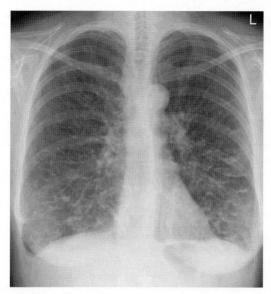

Fig. 4.28 CXR of a middle-aged woman with dyspnoea and cough revealing multiple ring shadows throughout both lungs in keeping with widespread bronchiectasis.

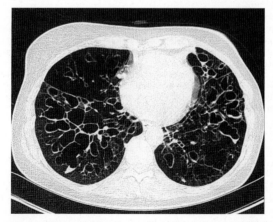

Fig. 4.29 Axial CT from the same patient as Fig. 4.28 better demonstrates the widespread bronchial dilatation, of both cystic and cylindrical type.

Cystic fibrosis

Definition

Cystic fibrosis is an autosomal recessive disease of epithelial transport which affects multiple organs, primarily lung, pancreas, GI tract, liver, and exocrine glands.

Clinical presentation

The majority of patients present in the 1st year of life with failure to thrive, recurrent respiratory infections, or meconium ileus at birth.

The dominant clinical picture and the major cause of mortality is progressive lung disease.

Respiratory

Patients have bronchiectasis with chronic cough and recurrent respiratory infections. Sinusitis and nasal polyps may be a feature. Clubbing may occur.

Gastrointestinal

- Pancreatic insufficiency may lead to steatorrhoea and malnutrition.
- Thick secretions can cause obstruction due to meconium ileus at birth, meconium ileus equivalent in older children, or intussusception. Fibrosing colonopathy is another cause of bowel obstruction.

Hepato-biliary

In some patients increased biliary viscosity results in cholestasis and eventually cirrhosis. This may present with jaundice or symptoms of portal hypertension such as bleeding from oesophageal varices.

Genitourinary tract

Male infertility is a frequent complication.

Imaging

Plain film

This is the mainstay of radiological evaluation in cystic fibrosis, used in routine screening and to detect complications. Progressive features include hyperinflation, bronchiectasis predominantly in upper zones with areas of mucus plugging and atelectasis.

Complications include infective consolidation, allergic bronchopulmonary aspergillosis (signs include bronchial dilatation with mucoid plugging—'finger in glove' sign) and pulmonary arterial hypertension (large central pulmonary arteries with peripheral pruning).

CT

- CT scanning is used as an adjunct to chest radiography and detects more changes of mucoid impaction and bronchiectasis.
- CT of the abdomen may have a role in the detection of complications such as the varied causes of bowel obstruction.

Ultrasound

Used in routine review of cystic fibrosis patients. The primary reason for surveillance is to detect portal hypertension which can occur secondary to biliary fibrosis. Other ultrasound features include a small echogenic pancreas and gallstones.

Information for the radiologist

- Obviously a known diagnosis of cystic fibrosis is essential on the request card or any previously documented complications.
- Previous imaging is essential for comparison of surveillance scans.

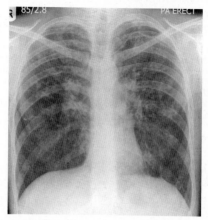

Fig. 4.30 PA CXR showing overexpanded lungs and upper lobe bronchiectasis typical of cystic fibrosis. Note in dwelling venous access device via the left arm.

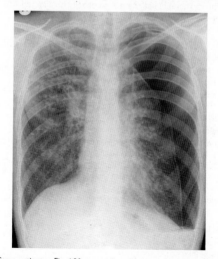

Fig. 4.31 Same patient as Fig. 4.30, presenting with acute shortness of breath. CXR now shows a large left pneumothorax with depression of the hemidiaphragm implying a tension pneumothorax. Treated with chest drain.

Pleural effusion

Pleural effusions are categorized as either transudates or exudates:
- Transudate protein level <30g/L.
- Exudate protein level >30g/L.

Transudates are caused by alterations to hydrostatic, colloid, or oncotic pressures in conditions such as cardiac failure, nephrotic syndrome, and liver failure.

Exudates are associated with inflammation of the pleura or subpleural lung parenchyma and are seen in infection, malignancy, or lung infarction.

In general exudative effusions require more evaluation and treatment.

Clinical presentation
- 15% of patients will be asymptomatic. When present symptoms include dyspnoea, non-productive cough, and pleuritic chest pain.
- Signs include dullness to percussion, decreased tactile fremitus, decreased breath sounds, and a pleural friction rub.

Imaging
Plain film (Fig. 4.32)
- Pleural fluid is not visualized on PA radiograph until >300ml are present.
- Lateral radiographs are better at detecting small effusions and can detect as little as 25ml.
- Hemidiaphragm and costophrenic recesses are obscured.
- Meniscus-shaped upper surface with the lowest point in mid-axillary line.
- On supine radiograph, hazy increased opacity on affected side, which does not obscure bronchovascular markings.

CT
- CT chest with contrast should be performed in all patients with undiagnosed effusion, especially if unilateral.
- Nodular pleural thickening suggests malignancy, smooth pleural thickening is seen in benign conditions such as empyema.
- In transudative effusions the pleura should not be visible at all.
- May be other findings such as cardiomegaly, asbestos plaque, abdominal disease.

Ultrasound
- Ultrasound is used to identify and localize fluid prior to aspiration or drainage. It also may be used to guide pleural biopsy.
- NCEPOD (National Confidential Enquiry into Perioperative Deaths) have recently recommended all drainage of pleural effusions be ultrasound-guided.
- Ultrasound is better than CT at showing loculation and septae within an effusion.

Information for the radiologist
- Relevant medical history.
- Features of infection if present.
- Asbestos exposure.

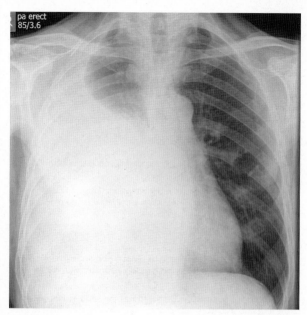

Fig. 4.32 PA CXR showing a large pleural effusion filling much of the right chest. Note the shift of the mediastinum away from the opacity and the meniscus extending up over the apex of the lung.

Interstitial lung disease

Inflammation of the supporting structures (interstitium) of the lung. Frequently results in scarring and fibrosis.

Clinical presentation

Common symptoms include dyspnoea and a dry cough. There may be clubbing and inspiratory crepitations on auscultation. A large number of causes are described including:

- Idiopathic, e.g. idiopathic pulmonary fibrosis (IPF), sarcoidosis.
- Inhaled substances, e.g. asbestosis, silicosis.
- Drug induced, e.g. amiodarone, gold.
- Infective causes, e.g. tuberculosis, atypical pneumonia.
- Connective tissue diseases, e.g. scleroderma, rheumatoid arthritis.
- Radiotherapy.

The diagnosis can often be made by integrating imaging findings with a detailed history, though occasionally bronchoalveloar lavage or lung biopsy is required.

Imaging

Plain film

Often abnormal with increased reticular ('linear') or reticular-nodular ('linear and nodular') lung markings. Fibrosis is usually associated with volume loss.

CT

HRCT is the preferred study. Demonstrates the smallest functional unit of the lung, the secondary pulmonary lobule, allowing abnormalities to be accurately localized.

Interstitial thickening is seen as either a reticular or reticular-nodular pattern.

Additional appearances may include:

- Honeycombing (small cystic spaces due to fibrosis).
- Nodules, e.g. in silicosis.
- Cysts, e.g. in histiocytosis.
- Bronchiectasis secondary to fibrosis (traction bronchiectasis).
- Lymphadenopathy, e.g. sarcoidosis, malignancy.
- Pleural plaques and calcification, e.g. asbestosis.

The distribution of disease is also important in narrowing the differential diagnosis, for example:

- Upper lobe predominance: TB, sarcoid.
- Lower lobe predominance: IPF, asbestosis, rheumatoid.
- Well-defined localized area: post-radiotherapy.

Information for the radiologist

- Presenting symptoms and duration of illness.
- History of malignancy/atypical infection/smoking.
- Potential environmental and drug causes, e.g. asbestos exposure.
- Lung function tests.

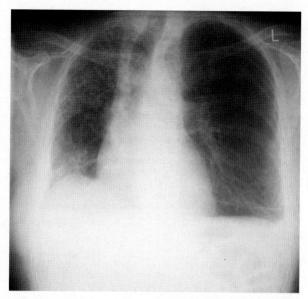

Fig. 4.33 PA CXR of a 60-year-old patient following a single lung transplant for idiopathic pulmonary fibrosis. Note the significant volume loss in the native fibrotic lung when compared to the transplanted left lung.

Connective tissue disease and the lung

Most of the connective tissue diseases (CTDs), including rheumatoid, systemic sclerosis, SLE, and dermatomyositis affect the lung in some way. Each condition has a different pattern of common effects, but there is considerable overlap between them.

Clinical presentation

Depends on severity of lung involvement and associated features of the underling disease. In many cases patients will present with lung involvement before any other manifestations of CTD.

Common symptoms are non-specific and include progressive exertional dyspnoea and dry cough. Haemoptysis occurs in patients with diffuse alveolar haemorrhage syndromes and vasculitis.

Chest pain is uncommon but pleuritic chest pain can occur in patients with rheumatoid arthritis or SLE.

Signs to look for include finger clubbing, a maculopapular rash, Raynaud's phenomenon, telangiectasia, peripheral lymphadenopathy, and inspiratory crackles on auscultation.

Imaging

Plain film (Fig. 4.34)
Rheumatoid lung
- Unilateral pleural effusion is a frequent manifestation.
- Fibrosis.
- Peripheral necrobiotic nodules.
- Bronchial wall thickening/bronchiectasis.
- Cor pulmonale: cardiac enlargement and pulmonary artery enlargement.

SLE
- Pleural and pericardial effusions.
- Non-resolving consolidation.

Systemic sclerosis
- Fibrosis.
- Oesophogeal dilatation.

CT (Fig. 4.35)
Shows the same features as CXR but in better detail with increased sensitivity and specificity.

Fluoroscopy
Barium swallow useful in assessing oesophageal dysmotility often seen in systemic sclerosis.

Information for the radiologist
- Duration of symptoms.
- Serological results.

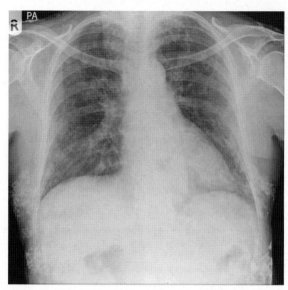

Fig. 4.34 CXR revealing widespread calcification within the soft tissues of the chest wall and distortion of the vascular pattern in the lung due to interstitial lung disease. The patient was proven to have dermatomyositis.

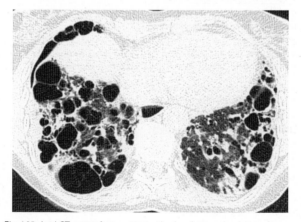

Fig. 4.35 Axial CT section from a patient with scleroderma and end-stage pulmonary fibrosis.

Pneumoconiosis

- The term pneumoconiosis refers to the accumulation of inorganic dust in the lungs and the tissue reaction to its presence.
- Silica, asbestos, coal, and beryllium are the most commonly encountered causes, usually inhaled during occupational exposure.
- The most important factors in the development of pneumoconiosis are the duration and intensity of exposure to the dust.

Clinical presentation

- Patients with simple coal worker's pneumoconiosis are usually asymptomatic. They may rarely report cough or sputum production.
- Complicated coal worker's pneumoconiosis (CWP) produces cough, dyspnoea, and lung function impairment. In advanced disease, cor pulmonale may result.

Imaging

Plain film (Fig. 4.36)

Simple CWP

- Small well-circumscribed nodules between 2–5mm with a predominant upper zone distribution.
- No progression after cessation of dust exposure.

Complicated CWP (progressive massive fibrosis, PMF)

- Large coalescent opacities >1cm.
- Typically peripheral in mid and upper zones: eventual hilar migration.
- May develop/progress after cessation of dust exposure.
- Calcified hilar lymphadenopathy.
- Loss of volume in upper zones.

Cavitation within the upper zone opacities may be seen due to ischaemic necrosis or possibly to superimposed TB.

CT (Fig. 4.37)

- Small well-defined nodules with upper zone predominance.
- Irregular conglomerate masses in both upper zones; may have cavitated.
- Focal centrilobular emphysema.
- Calcified mediastinal lymphadenopathy (peripheral calcification described as 'eggshell').

Information for the radiologist

- Respiratory function.
- Occupational history.
- Smoking history.
- Any worrying or unusual symptoms.

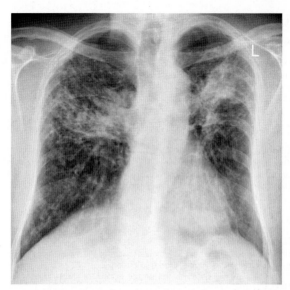

Fig. 4.36 PA CXR of patient with progressive massive fibrosis showing bilateral mass-like opacities at both hila, with volume loss in the upper lobes and widespread nodularity throughout the lungs, also with an upper lobe predominance. The patient had a long history of coal dust exposure.

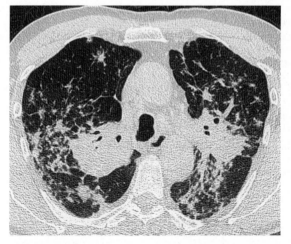

Fig. 4.37 Axial CT of the same patient as in Fig. 4.36, showing the bilateral mass-like lesions, nodularity, and architectural distortion of PMF.

Sarcoidosis

Sarcoidosis is a multisystem disorder of unknown cause. The diagnosis is usually made on the basis of wide ranging clinical and radiological manifestations, and is supported histologically by the presence of non-caseating granulomas. There is a worldwide distribution, although a geographic predilection for African American, Danish, and Swedish populations has been described. It typically affects young to middle-aged adults, with a slightly higher incidence in women.

Morbidity and mortality is usually related to pulmonary disease with a 1–5% fatality rate resulting from severe respiratory or cardiac dysfunction.

Clinical presentation

The clinical course of sarcoidosis varies considerably from self-limiting illness in up to 2/3 of patients, to chronic progression in 10–30% of cases. Dry cough, dyspnoea, and chest pain occur frequently.

Lofgren's syndrome is a form of sarcoidosis that manifests as fever, arthralgia, erythema nodosum, and bilateral hilar lymphadenopathy.

Imaging

Plain film (Fig. 4.38)

Findings include intrathoracic lymphadenopathy and parenchymal abnormalities often with an upper zone distribution.

A clinical staging system based on the pattern of chest radiographical findings is used to monitor disease progression and prognosis:

- Stage 0: normal chest radiograph.
- Stage 1: lymphadenopathy only.
- Stage 2: lymphadenopathy with parenchymal infiltration.
- Stage 3: parenchymal disease only.
- Stage 4: pulmonary fibrosis.

Ultrasound

Little routine role but used to assess abdominal involvement and aid biopsy of accessible nodes.

CT (Fig. 4.39)

Thoracic involvement is more clearly demonstrated than with CXR alone. CT will show the pattern of mediastinal involvement and subtle abnormalities such as pleural nodularity and bronchovascular thickening.

MRI

May be useful in cases of cardiac and neurological involvement.

Information for the radiologist

- Presenting features.
- Any concerns for alternative diagnoses such as TB or lymphoma.
- Serum ACE.

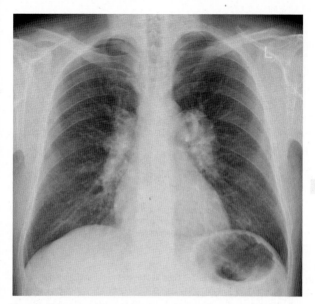

Fig. 4.38 CXR showing bilateral hilar adenopathy secondary to sarcoidosis.

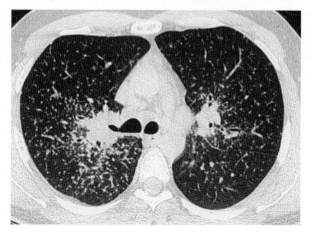

Fig. 4.39 Axial HRCT slice of patient with Sarcoid showing perihilar nodularity, thickening of the bronchovascular structures, and beading of the fissures.

Benign asbestos-related disease

Asbestos is a naturally occurring, fibrous silicate and exposure primarily occurs in occupational settings. The spectrum of asbestos-related thoracic diseases includes benign and malignant pleural disease:

- Benign pleural effusions are the earliest sign of disease (with a latency period of 8–10 years after exposure), and are usually small unilateral exudates.
- Focal pleural plaques are the radiological hallmark of prior asbestos exposure, and may or may not calcify.
- Diffuse pleural thickening is smooth and uninterrupted, involving the visceral pleura and extends over at least 25% of the chest wall.
- Round atelectasis specifically refers to an area of atelectatic lung adjacent to pleural thickening.
- Asbestosis is a term reserved for fibrosis due to asbestos exposure.

Clinical presentation

Patients are usually asymptomatic but asbestos effusions can present with episodes of pleuritic chest pain and fever. Diffuse pleural thickening may be sufficient to restrict chest movement and lead to breathlessness.

Imaging

Plain film (Fig. 4.40)

- En face calcified plaques are seen as well-defined opacities with irregular margins, sometimes describes as resembling a 'holly leaf'.
- Diffuse pleural thickening causes blunting of the costophrenic angles, is ill defined, and more extensive in distribution than focal plaque disease.
- Asbestosis manifests as pulmonary fibrosis in the basal, subpleural zones along with calcified plaque.

CT (Fig. 4.41)

Benign pleural plaques are focal, smooth opacities, usually <1 cm thick, paralleling the chest wall, often adjacent to ribs. The anterior chest and paravertebral positions are commonly affected sites. Calcification is common but not obligatory. The overlying lung is normal as the visceral pleura is unaffected.

Diffuse pleural thickening is more extensive and less well defined, normally seen in the paravertebral position. The overlying lung is affected as the viscera pleura contracts.

Round atelectasis has a characteristic appearance of a pleurally based mass, with indrawing of adjacent vessels and bronchi.

Asbestosis results in similar appearances to idiopathic fibrosis but with associated pleural disease.

Information for the radiologist

- Length and duration of asbestos exposure.
- Any features to suggest pleural malignancy, such as chest wall pain?

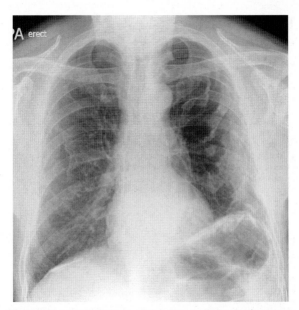

Fig. 4.40 CXR showing multiple areas of dense pleural calcification in keeping with asbestos plaque. Note how many plaques follow the line of the ribs, and the heavy diaphragmatic involvement.

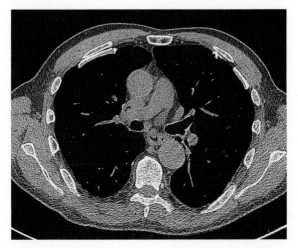

Fig. 4.41 Axial CT slice through typical, well-defined calcified pleural plaque on the anterior chest wall bilaterally.

Tuberculosis

- Tuberculosis (caused by *Mycobacterium tuberculosis*) remains the leading cause of death from infectious disease worldwide.
- Susceptible groups include the immunocompromised, infants, diabetics, and alcoholics.
- Frequency is increasing, especially amongst those with HIV infection.
- It is usually transmitted through inhalation. The organisms are deposited in the middle and lower lung zones, spread via the lymphatics to the hilar lymph nodes and then through the bloodstream to more distant sites such as the bone marrow, liver, spleen, kidneys, bones, and brain.
- After initial infection mycobacteria can remain dormant for many years, only causing clinical infection again when host immunity becomes impaired.
- Primary TB refers to disease at the site of initial deposition of mycobacteria in lung.
- Postprimary (or secondary) TB is caused by reactivation of dormant organisms.

Clinical presentation
- Cough.
- Weight loss/anorexia.
- Fever.
- Night sweats.
- Haemoptysis.
- Genitourinary symptoms; dysuria, hematuria, prostatitis, orchitis, and epididymitis may be present.
- Joint pain and swelling.

Altered mental status, neck stiffness, decreased level of consciousness, and raised intracranial pressure can indicate tuberculosis meningitis.

Imaging
Plain film (Fig. 4.42)
Primary TB
- Mediastinal lymphadenopathy: usually unilateral and more frequent in children.
- Consolidation.
- Ghon focus: calcified lung lesion.
- Ranke complex: Ghon focus + calcified lymph node.

Post-primary TB
- Consolidation in apical and posterior segments of upper lobes.
- Cavitation.
- Multifocal nodular opacities suggest 'miliary' TB.
- Occasionally present with unilateral effusion.

CT
- More sensitive and specific than plain film.
- Often shows signs of upper lobe volume loss, calcification and fibrosis in patients with previous (non-active) infection.

- Cavitations in a nodule or consolidation suggests active disease.
- Involved nodes classically show signs of central necrosis.
- Linear branching opacities and centrilobular nodules i.e. 'tree in bud' suggests endobronchial infection.

Ultrasound
- May be used to guide nodal biopsy or pleural aspiration.
- Useful in cases of renal or bladder involvement.

MR
Required if CNS involvement suspected.

Information for the radiologist
- Risk factors.
- Immune status.
- Bronchoscopy results if available.
- Treatment history.
- Vaccination history.

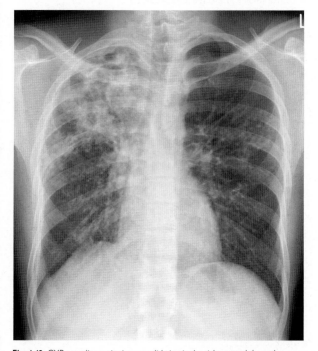

Fig. 4.42 CXR revealing cavitating consolidation in the right upper lobe and peribronchial thickening around the hilum on the left. TB infection was proven from sputum cultures.

Malignant pleural disease

Most malignant pleural effusions are metastatic. Common primaries to consider include breast, lung, and renal cancer.

Mesothelioma is the most common primary neoplasm of the pleura. Around 80% of cases of malignant mesothelioma are associated with previous asbestos exposure. The latency period between onset of exposure and development of mesothelioma is between 20–40 years.

Clinical presentation
- Insidious onset of dyspnoea, fatigue, weight loss.
- Chest pain is a worrying symptom.
- Signs of pleural effusion.

Imaging
Plain film
- Unilateral pleural effusion.
- Loss of volume in affected hemithorax.
- Rib destruction.

CT (Fig. 4.43)
CT chest with contrast should be performed in all patients with suspected pleural malignancy.

Signs on CT which are suggestive of pleural malignancy include:
- Irregular or nodular pleural thickening.
- Circumferential pleural disease, involving the mediastinal surface.
- Pleural thickening of >1cm.

CT can suggest pleural malignancy but is not in itself diagnostic, nor can it differentiate accurately between mesothelioma or metatstic pleural disease.

It may be used to perform targeted pleural biopsy.

MRI
Limited role—sometimes used if surgical resection being considered but this is rare.

Nuclear medicine
- PET-CT is not routinely used in mesothelioma unless curative surgery is being considered.
- Can be useful in cases of metastatic pleural malignancy of unknown primary.

Information for the radiologist
- Asbestos history.
- Any previous malignancy.

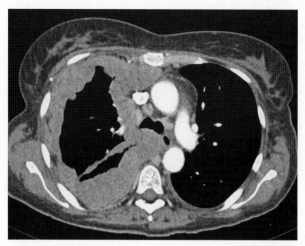

Fig. 4.43 Axial CT slice from a patient who presented with shortness of breath and right-chest pain. The scan reveals pleural thickening of >1cm in depth completely encasing the lung. Biopsy confirmed mesothelioma.

Mediastinal masses

An abnormal soft tissue mass within the mediastinum.

Clinical presentation

Wide range of presentations depending on location and nature of the mass. May present with chest pain, stridor, dyspnoea, dysphagia, SVC obstruction, hoarse voice, weight loss, back pain, or ruptured aneurysm, for example. May also be an incidental finding.

Imaging

Plain film (Fig. 4.44)

PA and lateral chest radiographs may identify and localize the mass and can help to guide further investigation.

CT (Fig. 4.45)

Usually performed for characterization and occasionally to guide biopsy. Identifies calcification, cystic areas, and vascular structures better than plain film. Allows accurate localization of the mass which narrows the differential diagnosis:

- Anterior mediastinum—anterior to the pericardium, 'the 4 T's':
  - Thymoma.
  - Thyroid.
  - Teratodermoid (germ cell tumours).
  - 'Terrible' lymphoma.
- Middle mediastinum—the heart, aortic root and pulmonary vessels:
  - Bronchogenic cysts and tumours.
  - Ascending aortic aneurysm.
  - Lymphadenopathy.
- Posterior mediastinum—posterior to the pericardium:
  - Oesophageal tumour, achalasia, or duplication cysts.
  - Descending aortic aneurysm.
  - Neurogenic tumour.
  - Meningocoele.
  - Extramedullary haematopoiesis.

Nuclear medicine

Certain tumours show increased uptake on PET, e.g. lymphoma. Scintigraphy can be used to identify thyroid goitre, ganglioneuromas and phaeochromocytomas.

MRI

Excellent at depicting neurogenic tumours and spinal abnormalities.

Ultrasound

Useful to assess the thyroid though will not visualize retrosternal areas adequately.

Information for the radiologist

- Age and sex of patient.
- Presenting symptoms.
- Previous imaging.
- Management plan, e.g. biopsy.

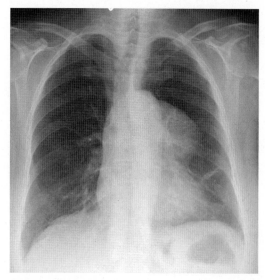

Fig. 4.44 PA CXR showing a large soft tissue mass arising from the mediastinum. Note the descending aorta is well seen, as are the hilar structures, placing the mass within the anterior mediastinum.

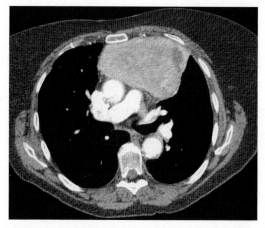

Fig. 4.45 CT of the same patient as Fig. 4.44, confirming the mass lies within the anterior mediastinum, enhances with contrast and contains some peripheral necrosis. CT-guided biopsy confirmed thymoma.

Vascular differential diagnosis

Global cardiomegaly

- Ischaemia.
- Cardiomyopathy.
- Pericardial effusion.
- Multiple valvular disease.

Enlarged left atrium

- Increased pressure:
  - Mitral stenosis.
  - Atrial myxoma.
  - Left ventricular failure.
- Increased flow:
  - Mitral incompetence.
  - Right-to-left shunt.

Enlarged left ventricle

- Increased pressure:
  - Hypertension.
  - Aortic stenosis.
  - Coarctation.
- Increased flow:
  - Aortic incompetence.
  - Mitral incompetence.
  - Right-to-left shunt.
- Weakened muscle:
  - Ischaemia.
  - Cardiomyopathy.

Enlarged thoracic aorta

- Aortic stenosis:
  - Post-stenotic dilatation of ascending aorta.
- Atherosclerosis.
- Hypertension.
- Infection:
  - Syphilis.
  - Endocarditis.
- Coarctation.
- Marfan's syndrome.
- Dissection.
- Post traumatic.

Enlarged pulmonary arteries

Dilated pulmonary trunk only
- Post-stenotic dilatation (pulmonary valve stenosis).

Dilated central pulmonary arteries/small peripheral vessels
- Primary pulmonary hypertension.
- Chronic pulmonary embolic disease.
- Chronic lung disease.
- Eisenmenger's syndrome.

Dilated central and peripheral vessels
- Left-to-right shunt.

Vascular presenting syndromes

Intermittent claudication

When atheroma narrows the blood vessels supplying the lower limb, blood flow is reduced and with it the amount of oxygen that can be taken up by the tissues.

Presentation

Muscle ischaemia presents in the same basic way, whether it be cardiac (angina) or in the lower limb (claudication). Patients suffer pain induced by exercise, relieved by rest. In claudication the pain is typically felt in the calves, and is brought on by walking.

Risk factors include:
- Increased age.
- Smoking.
- Hypertension.
- Family history.

Imaging

Ultrasound

Doppler ultrasound can be used in clinic to assess the patency of peripheral vessels, and follow up treated areas, but is not accurate enough to be used as a sole presurgical assessment.

CT

Can be used to visualize the peripheral vascular tree, but the radiation dose is high, and most centres prefer to use MRI.

MRI

Allows accurate assessment of the peripheral vasculature, identifying stenoses and occlusions in the main lower limb vessels down to the foot. Routinely used in the work-up of patients with claudication to plan intervention and follow-up patients after treatment.

Angiography

Diagnostic angiography has largely been superseded by MRI, but interventional radiologists have an ever increasing role in the treatment of these patients.

Rest pain

Once blood flow to the foot becomes critical, oxygen supply cannot match demand even at rest and the patient suffers continual pain in the lower limb.

Imaging techniques are the same as for claudication.

Acutely painful blue leg

Sudden occlusion of an artery results in acute ischaemia of the structures in that vascular territory. The commonest cause is thrombus, but cases can be iatrogenic, traumatic, or due to other embolic phenomena.

Presentation

Patients present with an acutely swollen, painful, pulseless leg. Capillary refill will be reduced and the limb is cold to the touch.

Risk factors include:
- Atrial fibrillation.
- Atheroma elsewhere, particularly the aorta.
- Smoking.

Imaging

Plain film

Little acute role but CXR may reveal cardiomegaly as a clue to an underlying cardiac cause.

Ultrasound

Echo should be performed to look for intra-cardiac thrombus, shunts, and valvular vegetations.

Peripheral Doppler ultrasound can be used to confirm the clinical impression of absent flow in the peripheral arteries.

CT

Can identify the level of occlusion, but more common role in the assessment of the aorta for atheromatous disease which may account for embolus formation.

MRI

Accurate localization of the site of thrombus and the condition of the rest of the peripheral vascular tree.

Angiography

In classic cases may still be used as the frontline diagnostic test, but this role now often given over to MRI. Angiography does allow catheters to be placed directly against the causative thrombus however, allowing intra-arterial thrombolysis to be administered, or other mechanical treatments if appropriate.

Vascular conditions

Aortic dissection

Dissection occurs when blood is able to track between the layers of the vessel wall, creating a false lumen beneath the intima.

Dissection is associated with hypertension, some connective tissue diseases, or may be iatrogenic.

Clinical presentation

Acute dissection will cause pain, often with associated neurological abnormalities or pulse and blood pressure inequalities. Classically the pain is described as having a 'tearing' quality, between the shoulder blades.

Aortic dissection classification and treatment depends on whether or not the ascending aorta is affected:

- Type A dissection involves the aorta proximal to the origin of the left subclavian artery and normally requires surgical treatment.
- Type B dissection only involves the aorta distal to the left subclavian and is commonly treated medically with antihypertensives.

Imaging features

Plain film

CXR is often normal. Classical findings in dissection include:

- Widened mediastinum or aortic arch.
- Tracheal deviation.
- Depression of the left main bronchus.
- Left pleural effusion.

Ultrasound

TOE can be used to diagnose thoracic aortic aneurysms and dissections at the bedside; however, it is highly operator dependent, less accurate than CT, and not readily available in many centres.

CT

Contrast-enhanced CT is the modality of choice for making the diagnosis and demonstrating the relevant anatomy. Allows accurate visualization of the dissection flap (Figs. 7.1 and 7.2), true and false lumens, and affected branches.

May demonstrate haemorrhage into the aortic wall, a sign of impending dissection and managed in much the same way.

CTA required for assessment prior to percutaneous stent placements.

MRI

Long procedure time and requirement for specialist (non-magnetic) monitoring equipment severely limits its role in acutely unwell patients.

Fluoroscopy

No role in acute diagnosis, however endovascular stents may be used to treat dissection flaps in the descending aorta.

Information for the radiologist

- Time since onset of symptoms.
- Blood pressure in both arms.
- Signs of shock.
- Previous history or risk factors for aneurysm.

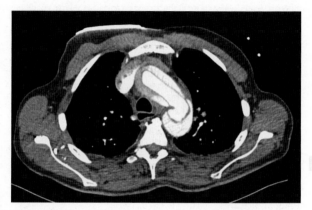

Fig. 7.1 Axial CT slice through the aortic arch in a patient presenting acutely with severe chest pain and signs of cardiovascular shock reveals a large dissection flap extending the length of the arch.

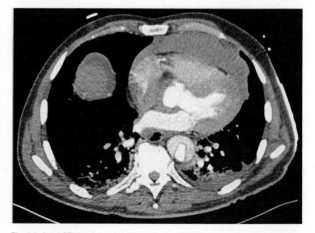

Fig. 7.2 Axial CT slice from the same patient as Fig. 7.1 at the level of the aortic root reveals a large pericardial effusion secondary to haemorrhage. Note also the dissection flap in the descending thoracic aorta.

Thoracic aneurysm

An aneurysm is present when the vessel diameter exceeds 150% of normal. Thoracic aneurysms may be secondary to atherosclerosis, infection, inflammation, or trauma.

Aneurysms of the arch and descending aorta are usually secondary to atherosclerosis, whilst those in the ascending aorta are seen in conditions such as aortic valve stenosis or Marfan's syndrome.

Risk of rupture increases with size, and is greater for aneurysms of the descending aorta than the ascending aorta.

Clinical presentation

- Many patients with thoracic aneurysms will be asymptomatic, diagnosed incidentally during investigation of other conditions.
- Ascending aortic aneurysms may involve the aortic root causing aortic regurgitation and congestive cardiac failure.
- Compression of local structures may cause wheeze or breathlessness (trachea), hoarseness (left recurrent laryngeal nerve) or dysphasia.
- Rupture occurs most commonly into the left pleural space and presents with pain, hypotension, and shock.
- Thromboembolism is another potential complication, causing stroke, lower limb ischaemic or mesenteric ischaemia. Symptoms will depend upon the area affected.

Imaging features

Plain film

Ascending aortic aneurysm may not be visible on plain film, or may give a bulge to the right mediastinum. The presence of curvilinear calcification in the aortic wall may be an indication of underlying aneurysm formation.

Ultrasound

TOE can be used to diagnose thoracic aortic aneurysms at the bedside; however, it is highly operator dependent, less accurate than CT, and not readily available in many centres.

CT

Contrast-enhanced CT is the modality of choice for making the diagnosis, demonstrating the relevant anatomy and is the modality of choice if acute rupture is suspected (Fig. 7.3).

CT is also used for accurate assessment prior to percutaneous stent placement.

MRI

Can be used to evaluate thoracic aneurysms, and allows interrogation of the aortic valve if post-stenotic dilation or aortic regurgitation are factors.

If long-term follow-up is required, allows accurate assessment without the radiation burden of CT.

Long procedure time and requirement for specialist (non-magnetic) monitoring equipment severely limits its role in acutely unwell.

Fluoroscopy
No role in acute diagnosis, however endovascular management of thoracic aortic aneurysms is now commonplace.

Information for the radiologist

- Time since onset of symptoms.
- Blood pressure in both arms.
- Signs of shock.
- Previous history or risk factors for aneurysm.

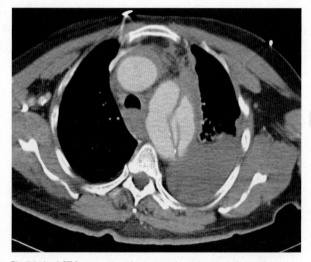

Fig. 7.3 Axial CT from a patient who presented acutely with cardiovascular compromise, revealing active haemorrhage from an aneurysm of the proximal descending aorta, with blood accumulating in the left chest. The patient died in the CT suite.

Acute myocardial infarction

Acute myocardial infarction (MI) is caused by sudden occlusion of a coronary artery leading to ischaemia and death of cardiac myocardium. Risk factors include increasing age, previous ischaemic heart disease, cigarette smoking, diabetes, hypertension, and hypercholesterolaemia.

Clinical presentation

Central chest pain is the sine qua non of acute myocardial infarction. The pain is usually centred over the lower left hemithorax, radiating to the left shoulder, jaw, and left arm. However, features may be atypical and occasionally present as upper abdominal pain.

An ECG will usually demonstrate ST-T changes confirming the diagnosis.

A subset of patients present without any chest pain or ECG changes and the diagnosis is made based on serum troponin rise.

Apart from intrathoracic conditions such as aortic dissection, pulmonary embolism, pneumonia, reflux oesophagitis, and pleural effusion, upper abdominal diseases such as peptic ulcer exacerbation, acute cholecystitis, and perforation peritonitis may all mimic an acute MI.

Imaging

Traditionally, imaging used to be of limited value in the initial evaluation of acute MI. However, with the advent of primary percutaneous intervention (PCI) and 'triple rule-out', this is changing.

Plain film

Chest radiographs may be completely normal unless patient develops acute left ventricular failure.

Echocardiogram

May demonstrate:
- Regional wall motion abnormalities.
- Mitral insufficiency.
- Ventricular septal rupture.
- Pericardial effusion.

Measured ejection fraction (EF) will provide an indication of the effect of the MI on cardiac function, which has prognostic relevance.

Coronary angiography

With the advent of primary PCI, coronary angiography and left ventriculography are performed in the acute setting with a view to proceed to appropriate intervention. It is performed usually by puncturing a femoral or (if necessary) brachial artery.

Using highly selective catheters and under fluoroscopic guidance, the coronary ostia are selectively engaged and small volumes of contrast agent injected to demonstrate the coronary arteries and any occlusion or stenoses. This then acts as a road map for further intervention.

Nuclear medicine

No role in the imaging of acute MI.

Have a greater role in ischaemic heart disease (see 📖 Ischaemic heart disease, p. 118).

CT

CT scanning does not have an established role in the management of acute ST elevation MI.

However, research is continuing into the use of CT to investigate patients who present with acute chest pain without ECG changes of MI as it can be used to simultaneously assess the coronary arteries, aorta, and pulmonary arterial tree to exclude significant coronary artery disease, aortic dissection, and acute pulmonary embolism. At present this remains a specialized investigation and is not widely available.

Information for the radiologist

- Duration of symptoms.
- Risk factors.
- ECG changes.
- Blood results.
- Heart rate and rhythm.

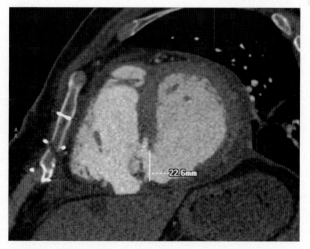

Fig. 7.4 CT reconstructed in the plane of the cardiac short axis in a patient with resistant heart failure following MI, demonstrating a post infarct VSD.

Cardiomyopathy

A structural or functional disease of heart muscle that is not secondary to ischaemia, valvular pathology, hypertension, or congenital abnormality.
  There are several distinct forms, including:

- Enlargement of the cardiac chambers (dilated cardiomyopathy, DCM).
- Hypertrophy of the cardiac muscle (hypertrophic CM, HCM).
- Loss of elasticity in the ventricle and reduced capacity to expand (restrictive CM, RCM).

Clinical presentation

- Clinical presentation is variable and includes fatigue, dyspnoea, chest pain, palpitations, and syncope.
- Diagnosis may occur through investigation of other family members after a sudden death or newly confirmed diagnosis.
- Causes of DCM include myocarditis (viral and bacterial), pregnancy, alcohol, and muscular dystrophies.
- Autosomal dominant inheritance is found in HCM; however, 50% of cases are sporadic.
- Examination findings include a displaced or forceful apex beat (in DCM and HCM respectively).
- HCM is associated with an ejection systolic murmur.
- Kussmaul's sign (elevation of JVP on inspiration) is found in RCM.
- Progression leads to signs and symptoms of cardiac failure.

Imaging features

Plain film (Fig. 7.5)

- Cardiomegaly is present in DCM and is a late feature of HCM.
- Heart failure develops with progressive disease.

Ultrasound/echocardiography

DCM

- Diffuse 4-chamber dilatation.
- Poor systolic function with normal left ventricular wall (LV) thickness.

HCM

- Asymmetric or symmetric LV wall thickening.
- Systolic anterior motion of the mitral valve.

DCM and HCM are both associated with mitral valve regurgitation.

RCM

- Poor late diastolic filling of the left ventricle.
- Dilatation of the left atrium with normal systolic function.

CT

- Can assess muscle thickness and heart size.
- Non-calcified pericardium <3mm thick helps exclude constrictive pericarditis as a differential for RCM.

MRI

- Similar to CT in terms of anatomical detail but gives better idea of ventricular and valvular function (Fig. 7.6).
- MRI can also be used to identify amyloid deposition, sarcoidosis (high T2), and haemochromatosis (low T1 and T2) as causes of DCM.

Angiography

- Ventricular volumes are increased in DCM and reduced in HCM. EF can be assessed and ischaemic causes excluded.
- RCM causes rapid early diastolic filling and poor late diastolic filling.
- Finally endomyocardial biopsy can be obtained in order to confirm the diagnosis.

Information for the radiologist

- Clinical history, family history, and differential diagnosis including ECG and echocardiography findings are helpful.
- Electrolytes prior to contrast-enhanced CT.
- Heart rate and rhythm if gated studies being considered.
- Remember patients with pacemakers can't have MRI.

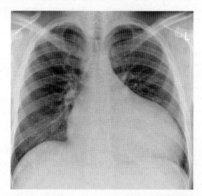

Fig. 7.5 PA CXR of a 23-year-old man presenting with dyspnoea revealing gross cardiomegaly. Echo confirmed enlargement of all 4 cardiac chambers in keeping with idiopathic cardiomyopathy.

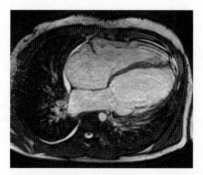

Fig. 7.6 Still image from a cardiac MRI study of the same patient as Fig. 7.5 revealing enlargement of all 4 cardiac chambers.

Coarctation of aorta

Coarctation is a localized narrowing of the aorta, normally occurring at the junction of the arch and descending thoracic aorta, resulting in an obstruction to blood flow.

Clinical presentation

Clinical presentation is dictated by the severity and extent of the narrowing, and features such as the presence of collateral vessels.

Severe coarctation can present with heart failure in the newborn. Associated cardiac anomalies such as patent ductus arteriosus (PDA) and ventricular septal defect (VSD) are common. Patients in whom the narrowing is less severe often present as older children or young adults with uncontrolled upper limb hypertension and weak femoral pulses.

The final subset is asymptomatic patients in whom coarctation is detected incidentally.

Imaging

Plain film (Fig. 7.7)

- In the neonatal group, the features are those of heart failure.
- The typical finding in the older age group is of a 'figure of 3' appearance of the proximal descending aorta.
- Bilateral rib notching seen on the under-surface of the ribs posteriorly is caused by enlarged intercostal arteries due to collateralization. It is best appreciated in the 3rd and 4th ribs.

Echocardiogram

Often the only imaging required in neonates, as it demonstrates:

- The coarctation segment, and its relationship with the ductus arteriosus.
- The pressure gradient across the narrowed segment.
- Associated cardiac anomalies.

In adults, the main value is to look for left ventricular hypertrophy (LVH) and associated anomalies such as bicuspid aortic valve.

CT (Fig. 7.8)

- Of value in adults who cannot undergo MRI.
- Gives excellent anatomical detail, but not the functional information of MRI.

MRI

Can provide anatomical detail, assess for intracardiac defects, and also provide information on the severity of the narrowing.

Angiography

With the increasing use of MRI, the diagnostic role of catheterization and angiography has reduced but is used therapeutically in cases where a balloon angioplasty or stent of the coarctation segment is possible.

Information for the radiologist

- Blood pressure difference between the 2 arms.
- Results of previous imaging such as echo.
- Detailed information regarding previous interventions and surgery.
- Details of the planned surgery.

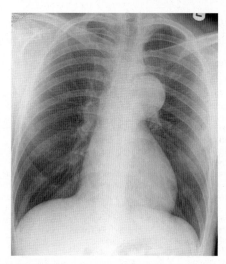

Fig. 7.7 PA CXR of a 20-year-old man presenting to A&E with an unrelated problem revealing marked focal dilatation of the aortic arch.

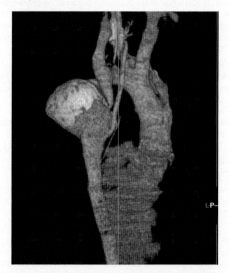

Fig. 7.8 Surface rendered CT image from the same patient as Fig. 7.7 demonstrating a tight, previously unsuspected coarctation with a large post-stenotic aneurysm of the aorta. Note the calcification in the aneurysm wall.

Aortic stenosis

Narrowing of the aortic valve (normal area 2.5–3.5cm^2) resulting in increased left ventricular work load and hypertrophy. Usually the valve area decreases to <1cm^2 before the patient becomes symptomatic.

Clinical presentation

Aortic stenosis (AS) is seen mainly in an elderly population as a consequence of degenerative disease in association with atherosclerosis. The other subset is younger patients, in whom the onset of stenosis is due to a congenitally bicuspid valve. Rheumatic involvement is uncommon in the Western world, but should still be considered in cases of multivalve disease.

Patients usually present with progressive exertional dyspnoea, syncopal attacks, chest pain, and heart failure.

Whilst valvular AS is by far the commonest cause, supravalvular stenosis (narrowing of the proximal ascending aorta in William's syndrome) and subvalvular stenosis (idiopathic hypertrophic subaortic stenosis) are alternatives and can be difficult to differentiate clinically.

Congenital bicuspid aortic valve leading to AS is associated with coarctation of aorta in conditions such as Turner's syndrome.

Imaging

Plain film

- Often normal although LCH and aortic valve calcification can be seen.
- Post-stenotic dilatation of the ascending aorta can be appreciated as a smooth prominence in the mid-right mediastinal outline (Fig. 7.9).
- Cardiomegaly is unusual, except when heart failure develops and its presence usually indicates mixed aortic valve disease or associated mitral valve disease.

Echocardiogram

Echocardiogram is the mainstay of diagnosis. It provides information on:
- The presence and severity of stenosis including the gradient across the aortic valve.
- Valve thickening and calcification.
- The effect on the left ventricle (wall thickness and chamber volumes).
- Associated valvular heart disease.

It is often useful in differentiating valvular AS from both the supravalvular and subvalvular types.

MRI (Fig. 7.10)

Little advantage over echo in most cases, however it is useful in patients with subvalvular stenosis to help identify the site, extent, and severity of stenosis and guide intervention.

CT

Little role in the assessment of valve function or stenosis but can exclude coexisting coronary artery disease, and is also useful in assessing aortic calcification prior to newer endovascular valve replacement techniques.

Angiography

Most patients with AS undergo cardiac catheterization for assessment of severity of disease and to exclude significant coronary artery disease.

Information for the radiologist
- Clinical presentation.
- Presence of other valvular disease, especially mitral disease.
- Previous imaging details to look for progression of disease.

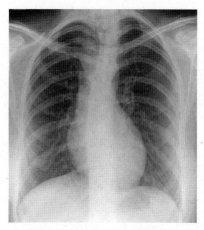

Fig. 7.9 CXR from a middle-aged man with dyspnoea. The curve of the cardiac apex suggests LVH and the ascending aorta is dilated.

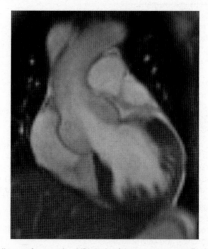

Fig. 7.10 Still image from cardiac MRI study of the same patient as Fig. 7.9 obtained in a plane to allow assessment of the aortic valve. Significant AS was confirmed.

Mitral valve disease

Mitral stenosis (MS), mitral regurgitation (MR), and mixed mitral disease represent the spectrum of mitral valve disease. Normal mitral valve area is between 4–6cm^2. Symptoms of MS develop once the valve area narrows to <2cm^2.

Clinical presentation

- Mitral valve disease presents with progressive dyspnoea.
- Patients with severe disease develop orthopnoea and paroxysmal nocturnal dyspnoea.
- Haemoptysis is a rare manifestation.
- Disease progression and physiological stress (e.g. pregnancy) may precipitate pulmonary oedema.
- Development of atrial fibrillation may result in worsening of symptoms.
- Patients are at risk of developing left atrial thrombus and associated thromboembolic complications.

Isolated mitral stenosis is usually due to rheumatic heart disease. Rarely it may be the result of valve involvement in carcinoid or collagen vascular disease and even more rarely a congenital malformation.

Mixed mitral disease is usually due to rheumatic heart disease.

MR has a much wider aetiology:
- It can develop acutely following rupture of a papillary muscle after MI or bacterial endocarditis.

Chronic MR may be due to:
- Stretching of the valve ring in patients with LV failure.
- Mitral valve prolapse.
- Myxomatous involvement.
- Rheumatic fever.
- Papillary muscle dysfunction with ischaemic heart disease.
- Congenital abnormalities of the mitral apparatus.

Imaging

Plain film

Signs of left atrial enlargement include:
- Double heart shadow.
- Splaying of carina (sub-carinal angle more than 75°).
- Elevation of left main bronchus.
- Enlargement of left atrial appendage (Fig. 7.11).

Progressive mitral valve disease will lead to pulmonary venous hypertension (see 📖 Left ventricular failure, p. 52).

Occasionally mitral valve calcification may be appreciated.

Rare features include ill-defined nodules (haemosiderosis) or densely calcified nodules in the middle or lower zones (pulmonary ossification).

Echocardiogram

Provides information about:
- The anatomy of the mitral valve and the subvalvular apparatus.
- Valve thickening and calcification.
- Mitral valve area.
- Papillary muscle status.

- Left atrial dimensions.
- Pulmonary hypertension and right ventricular function.
- Any associated cardiac abnormalities.

Further imaging is often not required.

The left atrium is the cardiac chamber closest to the oesophagus and TOE provides exquisite detail of the left atrium and mitral valve.

It is often used to look for signs of endocarditis and in theatre for the perioperative assessment of the mitral valve and the submitral apparatus.

MRI

- Occasionally in patients with previous surgery or congenital mitral disease MR may be performed to assess the intracardiac and major vascular anatomy (e.g. when MS is a part of hypoplastic left heart syndrome) but in general adds little to echo.
- Another role of cardiac MRI is in patients with ischaemic MR to assess myocardial viability.

Angiography

- Mainly reserved for patients >40 years or those with signs of associated ischaemic heart disease.
- Essential, however, as a part of percutaneous mitral valvotomy, prior to balloon valvotomy.

Information for the radiologist

- Clinical details including duration of symptoms.

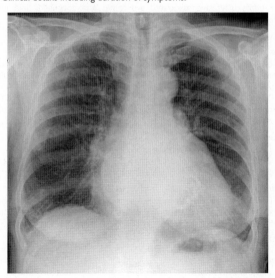

Fig. 7.11 PA CXR showing dense calcification of the mitral valve annulus and signs of left atrial enlargement—left atrial contour overlying the right heart, splaying of the carina, and enlargement of the left atrial appendage.

Congenital heart disease

This group of diseases include a wide spectrum of cardiovascular disorders of varying complexities and often associated with genetic syndromes and multisystem abnormalities. The age of presentation varies from before birth to adulthood depending on the nature of the abnormality.

Clinical presentation

CHD is broadly divided into 2 groups:
- Acyanotic lesions, which include left-to-right shunts such as atrial septal defect (ASD), VSD, PDA, and left-sided valvular diseases such as congenital MS and AS.
- Cyanotic lesions, which are typically right-to-left shunts such as tetralogy of Fallot or complex lesions leading to admixture of oxygenated and de-oxygenated blood such as total anomalous pulmonary venous drainage (TAPVD), truncus arteriosus, and single ventricle states.

Acyanotic lesions commonly present with failure to thrive, recurrent respiratory infections, 'attacks of asthma', and heart failure. If undetected they progress to pulmonary hypertension which may result in shunt reversal and the development of cyanosis (Eisenmengerization).

Cyanotic heart diseases typically present with cyanotic spells and failure to thrive. Those due to admixture lesions will often present with heart failure as well.

Patients may have associated syndromes and congenital anomalies affecting other organs and systems.

Imaging

Plain film (Fig. 7.12)

The CXR will not make a specific anatomical diagnosis, but combined with an appropriate history will allow broad categorization of disease and guide more specialized investigation.

Pulmonary plethora (increased vascular markings seen all the way to the periphery of the film) is seen in acyanotic heart disease. With progression of disease the lungs become darker and 'pruning' of the vessels is seen.

Echocardiography

- This is the mainstay of imaging for congenital heart disease.
- Outlines the anatomical abnormality and secondary changes such as chamber enlargement, wall hypertrophy, and cardiac function.

Cardiac catheterization

Using a peripheral (usually femoral) venous or arterial approach, allows assessment of cardiac anatomy, ventricular function, ventricular and pulmonary artery pressures.

Cardiac CT

- Has a limited but evolving role.
- May be used in patients with pacemakers or other metallic devices which preclude MRI.

- Provides useful anatomical detail but little functional information compared with echo or MRI.
- Advantages of CT over MRI include the demonstration of associated lung abnormality, speed of acquisition, and high spatial resolution.

Cardiac MRI

- Has an ever-expanding role, allowing assessment of:
  - Intra- and extracardiac anatomy.
  - Valvular function and pressure gradients.
  - Ventricular function and volumes.
- The lack of ionizing radiation is another advantage over CT in this group of patients, who are often young children needing follow-up imaging over a long period of time.

Information for the radiologist

- The suspected abnormality, echo results, exact information sought, and detail regarding previous intervention and surgery.
- It is important to know about pacemakers and metallic devices that preclude an MRI examination.

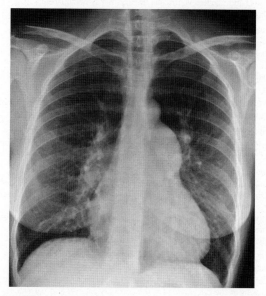

Fig. 7.12 CXR of an 18-year-old woman reveals marked enlargement of the pulmonary arteries, cardiomegaly, and plethoric lungs. Note also how the aortic arch appears smaller than usual. Echo confirmed a large ASD.

Ischaemic heart disease

A range of cardiac abnormalities caused by insufficient blood supply reaching the myocardial muscle mass, usually secondary to atherosclerotic narrowing of the coronary arteries. Associated with smoking, hypertension, diabetes, family history, hypercholesterolaemia.

Clinical presentation

May manifest acutely with severe central chest pain and breathlessness, either acute MI or unstable angina.

May have a more protracted course with occasional chest pain (angina) especially stress or exercise related, heart failure, ischaemic CM or cardiac arrhythmias.

Imaging

Plain film

- Chest radiographs may be completely normal.
- Cardiomegaly with left ventricular enlargement is often seen.
- Occasionally myocardial calcification due to a previous transmural infarct and calcified ventricular aneurysm may be apparent.
- May be signs of heart failure in the lung and pleural effusions.

Echocardiogram

Provides useful diagnostic and prognostic information including:

- Regional wall motion abnormalities.
- Chamber hypertrophy and enlargement.
- Identification of ventricular aneurysm and associated thrombus.
- EF.

It is valuable in follow-up after both medical treatment and percutaneous or surgical intervention.

Coronary angiography (Fig. 7.13)

Provides details of significant stenoses and occlusions in the coronary arteries and helps plan further percutaneous or surgical intervention.

Radionuclide perfusion studies

- Limited use in the acute setting but proven role in evaluating ischaemic damage to the heart and excluding ischaemia as a cause of non specific chest pain.
- Stress and rest Tl-201 and Tc99^m (MIBI scan) provides re-distribution information thus helping to identify viable but ischaemic muscle.
- MUGA scan using Tc-99^m labelled red blood cells can evaluate wall motion and EF.

Cardiac CT

- Calcium-scoring identifies the burden of coronary artery disease by looking at the calcium load in the coronary arteries and is useful in patients where the cause of chest pain is not established.
- CT coronary angiogram with contrast is not yet established as the modality of choice for imaging the coronaries prior to intervention but repeated studies show a high negative predictive value—i.e. is useful in excluding coronary artery disease.

ECG-gated MRI
- MRI has a tremendous potential in the imaging of ischaemic heart disease.
- Cine MRI is an accurate method of assessing cardiac function.
- Gadolinium-enhanced MRI can help identify areas of ischaemia, predict myocardial viability, and delineate areas of subendocardial infarction.

Information for the radiologist
- Duration of symptoms.
- Associated illnesses.
- Smoking history, medical history.
- ECG findings including cardiac rhythm.

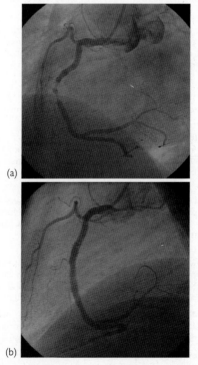

Fig. 7.13 (a) Coronary angiogram of a man with severe angina reveals a significant stenosis in the right coronary artery. (b) Same patient following endovascular stenting of the stenosis, which resulted in maintained symptom relief.

Cardiac tumours

Cardiac tumours may be primary or secondary. Metastatic disease from an extra cardiac tumour is the most common cause of an intracardiac mass. Lung and breast are the most common primary sites.

Primary cardiac tumours are rare and more often benign than malignant. Some of the more common primary tumours include:

- Myxoma: the most common primary cardiac tumour, and benign (Fig. 7.14). Usually occurs in left atrium, often arising from a 'stalk-like' pedicle.
- Lipoma.
- Rhabdomyoma: most common primary tumour in paediatric group, associated with tuberous sclerosis.
- Sarcoma: the most common primary malignant cardiac tumour is angiosarcoma but there are many other types of sarcoma.

Clinical presentation

Present at any age with palpitations, shortness of breath, cough, chest pain, or syncope. Clinically there may be a heart murmur, arrhythmia, or evidence of cardiac failure. May present with complications such as pulmonary emboli or endocarditis.

Imaging

Plain film

Rarely able to detect the tumour but may reveal cardiomegaly, left atrial enlargement, calcification, or pulmonary oedema.

Ultrasound (echocardiogram)

Usually the initial specialist investigation, offers real-time imaging of the tumour throughout the cardiac cycle and good anatomical detail. Provides information on cardiac and valvular function.

CT

Sensitive but often unable to characterize the mass. Modern 'ECG-gated' techniques provide excellent anatomical information. More commonly used to look for a primary tumour elsewhere if the cardiac mass is thought to be a metastasis.

MRI

More sensitive than echocardiography and unlike CT is radiation free. However, does require prolonged breath-holding which can be difficult for some patients. Depicts cardiac anatomy, ventricular and valvular function, and offers more information regarding tissue characteristics than CT.

Nuclear medicine

MIBG (metaiodobenzylguanidine) scans can detect phaeochromocytoma with high sensitivity. PET may be useful if metastatic disease is suspected.

Information for the radiologist

- History of malignancy.
- Concern for complications, e.g. heart failure, valvular disease, PE.
- Heart and respiratory rate/rhythm—affect suitability for MRI/CT.
- Echocardiogram findings.

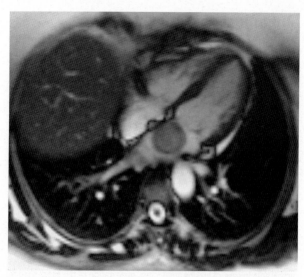

Fig. 7.14 Axial image from a cardiac MRI study revealing a soft tissue mass adherent to the wall of the left atrium. Surgery confirmed a left atrial myxoma.

Abdominal aortic aneurysm

Defined as widening of the aortic calibre to >3cm, or at least 1.5 times the calibre of an adjacent normal segment.

Clinical presentation

Clinical presentation varies widely. Often they are picked up incidentally on imaging such as an abdominal ultrasound. Occasionally, they present with symptoms such as pain or a palpable, pulsatile mass. Rarely, they can present as an acute emergency following active leak or rupture.

Up to 80% of aneurysms are fusiform with circumferential involvement. The remainder are saccular. True aneurysms involve all 3 layers of the wall, whilst pseudo-aneurysms (usually seen following trauma or previous limited dissection) are due to partial disruption of the aortic wall with the escaping blood limited by adventitia.

Aneurysms of the descending thoracic and abdominal aorta are usually the result of atherosclerosis. Although most common in the infra-renal aorta, various segments can be involved and occasionally extensive thoracoabdominal aneurysms may be seen.

Imaging

Plain film

The outline of a calcified aneurysm can be appreciated on the abdominal radiograph. In case of leaking aneurysms, obscuration of the psoas shadow may be seen.

Ultrasound

Abdominal ultrasound is the mainstay of aneurysm surveillance allowing accurate measurements of the aortic dimension (Fig. 7.15). Most patients with abdominal aortic aneurysm will have yearly ultrasound to look for increasing aneurysm size, which may eventually necessitate surgical repair.

CT angiogram

Multislice CT scanning is the investigation of choice if intervention is required, either surgical or radiological. Arterial phase imaging shows the exact extent of the aneurysm, branch involvement and identifies cases suitable for endovascular therapy (EVAR) (Fig. 7.16).

CTA is also used in the follow-up of EVAR to identify any post-procedural stent related complication.

When patients present acutely with suspected bleeding or leakage, urgent CT to confirm the diagnosis and plan best treatment is appropriate.

Contrast-enhanced MRI

There is a limited role for contrast-enhanced MRI in those patients where radiation exposure is a major issue or others with iodine allergy which precludes the use of CT contrast.

Information for the radiologist

Any previous imaging and documented measurements of the aneurysm and the treatment plan (surgery versus endovascular).

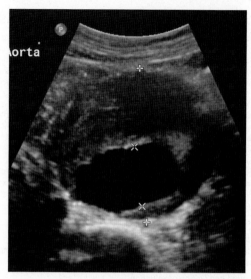

Fig. 7.15 Abdominal ultrasound image revealing a 5.6cm aneurysm of the aorta. Note how the thick layer of intramural thrombus is differentiated from the echo free vessel lumen.

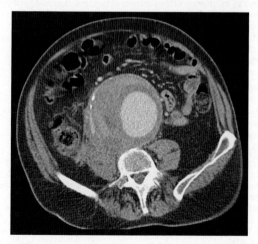

Fig. 7.16 CT scan from a different patient revealing a large aneurysm with signs of haemorrhage into the aneurysm wall and leak into the retroperitoneum. The patient went straight from CT to have an endovascular stent.

Peripheral vascular disease: diagnosis

A group of diseases of different aetiologies, affecting the arteries of the upper and lower extremities. Atherosclerosis is the predominant cause. Diabetes mellitus, hypertension, hypercholesterolaemia, smoking and age are major risk factors. Other causes include Buerger's disease, inflammatory and autoimmune arteritis, Raynaud's disease, and thromboembolism.

Clinical presentation

- Claudication is the hallmark of early peripheral vascular disease (PVD). It is a cramping muscular pain due that develops on exertion and is relieved by rest.
- Progression of disease leads to rest pain, non-healing ulcers, and occasionally gangrene.
- Patients with acute thromboembolism present with a painful white leg.
- Along with the clinical presentation, ankle–brachial pressure index (ABPI) (the ratio of the systolic pressure at the ankle to that in the arm) is used for risk stratification of patients with PVD.

Imaging

Plain film

This is of limited value in PVD. However, due to the common risk factors almost all patients should have a plain chest radiograph.

Ultrasound and Doppler evaluation

- This is a vital initial assessment tool of the peripheral vascular anatomy and identifies the site and severity of stenosis.
- Provides information of the location, extent, and morphology of the stenotic lesion.
- Doppler assesses the impact of the lesion on flow, the degree of turbulence created, post-stenotic velocity (which indicates the degree of obstruction), and the distal run-off.
- Ultrasound is also important in the follow-up of patients after treatment to identify those needing early re-intervention.

Angiography

As CT and MR develop, the role of diagnostic angiography is diminishing. However, it remains the 'gold standard' for assessing the anatomy and disease burden and is a part of the assessment prior to endovascular intervention (see 📖 Angiography, p. 6).

CT angiogram

- Current multislice CT scanners allow the imaging of the entire peripheral arterial tree without arterial catheterization (needed for angiography).
- Iodine-based contrast agent injected into a peripheral venous cannula is used to visualize the arteries.
- Spatial resolution is superior to that of MRI, but there is a significant radiation burden.
- CT is especially useful in heavily calcified arteries and in the presence of stents.

Whilst the images are acquired in the axial plane, modern scanners and computer software allows the vessels to be displayed in various ways:
- Multi-planar reformats (MPR) view the vessel along its course.

- Maximum intensity projection (MIP) picks the brightest pixel in each location and provides an angiogram like picture.
- Shaded surface display (SSD) utilizes the pixels on the surface.
- Volume rendering (VR) techniques combine SSD and MIP to provide a 3D image of the region of interest.

MR angiogram (Fig. 7.17)
- A gadolinium-enhanced MR study of the peripheral vascular tree.
- The various imaging manipulations such as MPR, MIP, and VR can all be used as for CTA.
- The two major advantages of MR over CT are the ability to image in different planes (e.g. along the length of the vessel) and the absence of any radiation burden.
- MRA is gradually becoming the investigation of choice in the assessment of PVD prior to intervention/surgery, except in cases where it is either contraindicated or technically limited (stents or heavy calcification).

Information for the radiologist
- Duration and level of symptoms, e.g. presence of rest pain.
- Pacemaker?
- Blood results including INR if arterial puncture being contemplated.
- Any previous imaging and intervention.

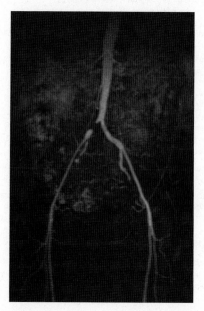

Fig. 7.17 Image from an MR angiogram revealing a tight focal stenosis in the right common iliac artery.

Peripheral vascular disease: radiological treatments

Endovascular intervention has revolutionized the management of PVD. New balloon catheters and stents provide the interventional radiologist with a wide armamentarium to tackle various lesions. The basic principle of endovascular intervention is the dilatation of a stenosed segment by applying a strong but controlled centrifugal force, which results in stretching and fissuring of the vessel and in time to remodelling. In specific instances, a tubular mesh (stent) is used as a scaffold to hold the segment open while remodelling occurs.

Indications
- Worsening claudication.
- Rest pain.
- Failed medical treatment.
- Significant stenosis (more than a 50% luminal compromise).

Stents are used in larger vessels or when balloon dilatation is either not practical or has failed.
   Relative contraindications include:
- The presence of long segment severe stenosis.
- Multiple severe narrowings affecting a long segment.
- Occluded segment.
- Contraindication to contrast (although either CO_2 or gadolinium may be used in cases of allergy to iodinated contrast).

Distal small vessel disease, affecting the foot vessels, is not treated endovascularly.

Different types of endovascular intervention
1 Balloon angioplasty.
2 Laser angioplasty and cryoplasty.
3 Atherectomy: directional and rotational types.
4 Stents: covered or bare-metal stents, self- and balloon-expandable stents, nitinol stents, drug-eluting stents, stent grafts.

Procedure
Consent
Informed consent should include the risk of access site complications, failure of procedure, vessel dissection, and distal embolization.

Access
The common femoral artery is most commonly used. Brachial route is occasionally needed.

Local preparation
The site is cleaned and local anaesthesia administered. Under strict asepsis the appropriate vessel is punctured with a suitable needle.

Technique
Once the vessel is punctured and a catheter is passed, an angiographic run is performed to outline the anatomy of the diseased segment and visualize

the run-off. These images are transferred to an adjacent screen to be used as a road map for the intervention.

The next stage is to pass a guidewire and a balloon catheter across the stenotic segment.

The balloon is connected to a pressure gauge (which helps guide the balloon dilatation) and gradually expanded until maximum dilatation is reached.

Following the procedure, a completion angiogram is performed to assess the outcome and also the run-off (Fig. 7.18).

The principles of stent dilatation are essentially the same. Stents may either be balloon-expandable or self-expandable.

Complications
- Puncture site complications: haematoma, pseudo-aneurysm, dissection, AV fistula, and infection.
- Contrast allergy and anaphylaxis.
- Stent migration, balloon and stent rupture.
- Distal embolization.

Information for the radiologist
- Renal function.
- Clotting profile.
- Prior imaging.
- Any major underlying morbidity.

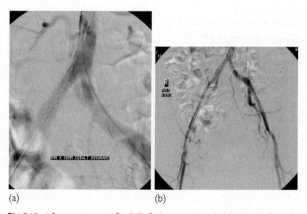

(a)   (b)

Fig. 7.18 a) Same patient as in Fig. 7.17. Catheter angiography has been performed and a metal stent placed across the iliac artery stenosis. b) Catheter angiography post-stent deployment confirms good flow of contrast into the peripheral vessels of both legs.

IVC filter insertion

Pulmonary embolism (PE) is a common and sometimes fatal complication of deep vein thrombosis (DVT). By insertion of a filter into the IVC, a mechanical obstacle is created in the path of any thrombus travelling up the IVC toward the heart.

Indications

An IVC filter may be permanent or retrievable, depending on the reason for insertion. Whilst controversy exists about the relative indications for filter insertion, their use is widely accepted in the following situations:

- DVT/PE in patients with a contraindication to anticoagulation such as a recent major intracranial bleed.
- Progression of venous thromboembolism despite adequate anticoagulation.

In selected situations, they may be inserted prophylactically.

- Floating iliac thrombus.
- Patients with major trauma and DVT.
- Patients with DVT who are to undergo major surgery.
- PE/DVT in pregnancy.

Procedure

Consent

Written informed consent including failure of deployment, migration of the filter, and thrombus forming on the device.

Access

Usually performed from a jugular or femoral approach.

Inferior venacavogram

Catheter in the low IVC and a flush injection to evaluate the IVC for clots and identify the renal vein origins.

Deployment

The filter is optimally deployed in the infrarenal IVC (Fig. 7.19), although on occasion they can be deployed above the renal veins.

Complications

- Related to the puncture site: bleeding, haematoma.
- Related to the filter: migration of the filter into the heart, tilted filter (may need deployment of another filter), filter thrombosis (potentially life threatening and may warrant removal).

Information for the radiologist

- Previous imaging.
- Infection status.
- Clotting status is vital before proceeding with the filter insertion.
- Clinical background and indication.

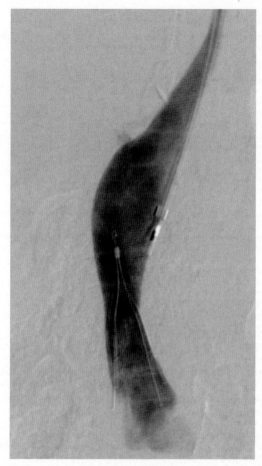

Fig. 7.19 Image acquired after deployment of an IVC filter confirms the position of the device in the IVC, below the level of the renal veins. Note the small hook on its top end to help with retrieval should that be appropriate.

Arteriovenous fistula

A connection between an artery and an adjacent vein which results in shunting of blood to the venous side bypassing the distal segment.

Aetiology
- Congenital: visceral or peripheral vascular.
- Syndromic: Osler–Rendu–Weber syndrome.
- Post-traumatic.
- Pathological processes such as infection or malignancy resulting in erosion of vessels and development of abnormal connections.
- Iatrogenic: following femoral punctures, visceral biopsies.
- Therapeutic: arteriovenous fistula (AVF) created surgically for haemodialysis.

Clinical presentation
- They are often asymptomatic.
- High-flow shunting can lead to high-output heart failure.
- A palpable thrill with an associated continuous murmur is the clinical hallmark of a peripheral fistula.
- Compression of peripheral AVF may result in bradycardia (Branham's sign).
- Local gigantism and vascular insufficiency distal to the fistulous connection are known sequelae.
- In the viscera, shunting can lead to distal infarcts and AVF in the lung can cause paradoxical embolism—these patients may present with CVA.
- Peripheral AVF, including those created for haemodialysis, result in arterialization of the veins (dilated, prominent, and tortuous).

Imaging
Plain film
Limited role, but pulmonary AV fistulae can have typical appearances—a pulmonary nodule with prominent feeding artery and draining veins.

Ultrasound and Doppler
- Peripheral and some visceral (e.g. renal) AVF are diagnosed on ultrasound/Doppler assessment.
- Colour Doppler demonstrates turbulence at the site of fistula.
- Pulsed Doppler adds information by demonstrating focal low resistance arterial flow with continuous forward flow throughout the cardiac cycle. It will also demonstrate the arterialized (pulsatile) trace of the venous waveform.

Ultrasound is invaluable in assessing surgical AVF in patients on dialysis for early detection of complications such as stenosis, thrombosis, and occlusion.

Venography (prior to formation of AVF)
Upper limb venography is essential to demonstrate the venous anatomy prior to formation of an AVF.

This is performed by segment-wise injection of the veins and imaging the forearm, arm, and proximal veins one after the other. For the proximal intrathoracic veins, simultaneous injection from both sides is required.

Radionuclide imaging

Some visceral AVF (such as pulmonary and hepatic) can be assessed using Tc-99m labelled sulphur colloid or macroaggregated albumin. This is occasionally required when clinical and Doppler assessments are equivocal about the degree of shunting.

CT and MR

Both CT and MRA can be used to identifying visceral AVF and their associated sequelae and complications (Fig. 7.20). HRCT is used to diagnose AVMs in the lung.

Information for the radiologist

- Any previous fistulae that have been created and subsequent complications or intervention should be conveyed when requesting a Doppler examination or venography.
- Clinical signs.
- Blood results, including O_2 saturations if large shunts are suspected.

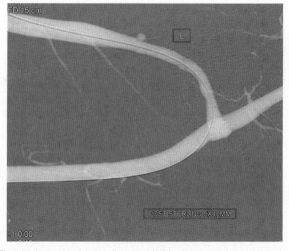

Fig. 7.20 Angiogram of a surgically created AVF for dialysis in a patient with renal failure. Note the wire crossing between the artery and vein which has been used to stretch a stenosis of the fistula.

Neurology differential diagnosis

Intracerebral 'mass'

- Primary brain tumour, e.g. glioblastoma multiforme.
- Metastasis.
- Arterial infarct.
- Abscess.
- Demyelination.
- Haematoma.
- Encephalitis.
- Aneurysm.

Intracranial calcification

- Normal structures:
  - Pineal gland.
  - Choroid plexus.
  - Dura.
  - Basal ganglia.
  - Arachnoid granulations.
- Vascular:
  - Atherosclerosis.
  - Aneurysms.
  - AVM.
  - Old infarct/haemorrhage.
- Tumours:
  - Commonly meningioma.
- Infections:
  - e.g. TB.
- Basal ganglia calcification:
  - Normal.
  - Endocrine.
  - Metabolic.
  - Infection.
  - Toxic.
- Neurocutaneous syndromes:
  - Sturge–Weber syndrome.
  - Tuberous sclerosis.
  - Neurofibromatosis.

Multiple-ring enhancing lesions

- Metastases.
- Abscesses.
- Lymphoma.
- Demyelination.
- Multifocal glioma.
- Multiple infarcts.
- Contusions/haematomas.

Cerebellopontine angle mass

- Acoustic neuroma.
- Meningioma.
- Epidermoid.
- Aneurysm.
- Metastasis.

Neurology presenting syndromes

Altered consciousness

Measured on the Glasgow Coma Scale, this can vary from mild confusion to coma.

Clues are often in the history to determine the cause, e.g. trauma/infective/toxic. Imaging may be urgently needed to identify surgically treatable causes, e.g. extradural haemorrhage in trauma patients.

- Infection:
  - Meningitis: bacterial/viral.
  - Encephalitis.
  - Empyema.
  - Intracerebral abscess.
- Haemorrhage (traumatic or spontaneous rupture, e.g. AVM):
  - Intra-axial: within the brain parenchyma.
  - Extra-axial: outside the parenchyma.
- Ischaemic:
  - Cardiorespiratory arrest.
  - Near drowning.
  - Hypovolaemia (important in trauma patients).
- Toxic:
  - Carbon monoxide poisoning.
  - Overdose, e.g. heroin.
- Metabolic:
  - Diabetic ketoacidosis.
  - Hepatic encephalopathy.
  - Renal failure.
  - Metabolic disorders.
- Tumour.
- Epilepsy (post ictal).
- Vascular:
  - Stroke.
- Demyelination disorders.

Role of imaging

CT
Useful in the acute setting, to exclude haemorrhage, space-occupying lesions, identify stroke, or evidence of established ischaemia.

Headache

The majority of patients with headaches do not require imaging. Worrying symptoms include signs of increased intracranial pressure such as headaches worsening on lying flat, bending down, or worsening daily headaches should be investigated. Headaches presenting acutely associated with meningism should be investigated immediately.

- Infection:
  - Meningitis.
  - Encephalitis.
  - Sinusitis.
- Haemorrhage:
  - Subarachnoid, intracerebral, or extra-axial.
- Post-traumatic.
- Raised intracranial pressure:
  - Brain tumours.
  - Idiopathic intracranial hypertension.
- Venous sinus thrombosis.

Role of imaging

CT

Useful in acute presentation, urgently if associated with meningism.

Neurology conditions

Stroke

Stroke is an acute episode of neurological deficit. Transient ischaemic attacks (TIAs) are neurological events that resolve within 24 hours (usually within 1–2 hours). Stroke is a major health problem in the UK accounting for 11% of annual deaths as well as significant morbidity.

Causes
- 80% thrombotic (cerebral infarction).
- 15% haemorrhagic.
- 5% non-traumatic subarachnoid haemorrhage (SAH).
- 1% venous occlusion.

Clinical presentation

Patients present with facial and limb weakness, slurred speech, numbness, blurred vision, confusion and headache. FAST (**F**ace **A**rm **S**peech **T**est) is used to rapidly screen patients.

110,000 people will suffer a first or recurrent stroke every year in England. Thrombolytic therapy is indicated for use in thrombotic stroke. This must be given within 3 hours of onset of symptoms once haemorrhage has been excluded. Realistically this will be within 6 hours of symptom onset within a specialized stroke unit.

Imaging

Ultrasound

Doppler ultrasound of the carotid arteries is used in patients with TIA or non-disabling stroke as part of the work-up for possible carotid endarterectomy. Carotid artery stenosis is calculated from assessing arterial flow rates. Symptomatic patients with stenoses >70% are considered candidates for endarterectomy.

CT (Fig. 10.1)

All patients with a suspected stroke should have a non-contrast CT (NCCT) of the brain within 24 hours. Immediate imaging (within 1 hour) is indicated in the following circumstances:
- Indications for thrombolysis or early anticoagulation treatment.
- Anticoagulant treatment.
- Known bleeding tendency.
- Glasgow Coma Score (GCS) <13.
- Unexplained progressive or fluctuating symptoms.
- Papilloedema, neck stiffness, or fever.
- Severe headache at symptom onset.

NCCT is used to exclude haemorrhage or other causes. Early NCCT in stroke is often normal. Initial findings include loss of grey/white differentiation, sulcal effacement, and a hyperdense (bright) clot within a major cerebral artery (the hyperdense MCA sign). Later, within 12–24 hours, oedema can be detected as low density within the brain parenchyma. Old/mature infarcts are hypodense (dark) on NCCT and associated with local atrophy.

MRI is more sensitive than CT in detecting oedema—within 6 hours, but is not as widely available in the acute setting. Oedema is seen as high signal on T2 and FLAIR imaging.

Intracerebral haemorrhage is seen as a high density (bright) focus on NCCT. This most often occurs secondary to hypertension, 80% are within the basal ganglia. The MRI appearance of haemorrhage differs according to the age of the blood products.

Various other techniques can be used in the imaging of stroke. These include: CTA, CT/MR perfusion studies, and diffusion weighted MRI. These will be used in specialist stroke centres and are not yet widely used in acute stroke imaging.

Information for the radiologist

An accurate history is vital to assess whether the patient is a candidate for thrombolysis or any of the other indications for immediate imaging (see earlier in section).

What are the patient's current clinical state and GCS? Patients who are confused can be uncooperative and difficult to scan. Patients with a low GCS may have difficulty protecting their airway and anaesthetic support may be required prior to scanning.

Patients with known malignancy may have intracranial metastases causing their symptoms. These are not always visible on NCCT and therefore a contrast enhanced CT scan may be indicated.

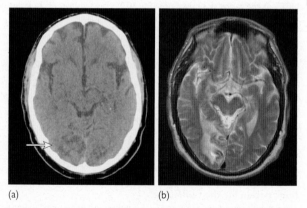

(a)   (b)

Fig. 10.1 A 77-year-old male with left visual disturbance. a) Axial CT image, the arrow shows an area of low attenuation. b) Axial T2 MRI showing the full extent of the stroke.

Subarachnoid haemorrhage

SAH is the presence of blood within the subarachnoid space, which can sometimes extend into the intraventricular space. Vasospasm and cerebral infarction is the leading cause of death in SAH.

Causes

- Rupture of cerebral aneurysm (90%).
- Trauma.
- Arteriovenous malformation (AVM).
- Coagulopathy.
- Extension of intracerebral haemorrhage.
- Idiopathic (5%).

Clinical presentation

Headache—sudden onset, worst ever, 'thunderclap', often radiating towards occiput. Neck stiffness and photophobia related to meningeal irritation by blood products are often present. Nausea, vomiting, confusion and decreased level of consciousness are symptoms related to raised intracranial pressure. Patients may present with symptoms related to complications such as hydrocephalus, vasospasm, and stroke.

Patients with a history of polycystic kidney disease, aortic coarctation, fibromuscular dysplasia, and collagen vascular disorders are at increased risk of cerebral aneurysm.

Imaging

NCCT is the mainstay of diagnosis (Fig. 10.2). It is sensitive (95%) in the first 24 hours. High-density (bright) blood can be seen in the basal cisterns, Sylvian fissure, ventricles, over the cortical sulci, or interhemispheric fissure. The site of the blood can point to the location of the ruptured aneurysm.

Hydrocephalus is an early complication and can be detected on CT as dilatation of the ventricles.

MRI is more sensitive than CT in detecting SAH in the subacute phase (after 48 hours) and chronic SAH. If imaging is negative then lumbar puncture is required to confirm the diagnosis.

Further imaging is directed at identifying the underlying cause. CTA is as accurate in diagnosing cerebral aneurysms as standard catheter angiography. This is readily available in most centres, is non-invasive, and can be performed immediately following the diagnostic NCCT.

Most cerebral aneurysms can be treated endovascularly by the placement of coils.

Information for the radiologist

The patient's clinical condition and GCS is important. Anaesthetic support may be required.

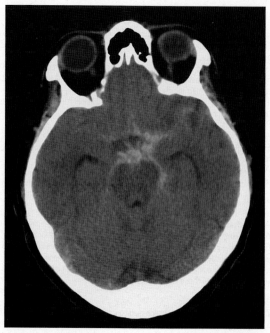

Fig. 10.2 Axial non-contrast-enhanced CT image showing extensive subarachnoid haemorrhage (the central white areas).

Subdural haemorrhage

Subdural haemorrhage (SDH) is the presence of blood within the subdural space. These are usually secondary to tears in the emissary veins as they cross the subdural space.

Acute SDHs have a high associated mortality due to the fact that they are usually secondary to high-energy acceleration/deceleration mechanisms with a high incidence of other injuries.

They can cause an increase in the intracranial pressure with brain tissue injury being the result.

Predisposing factors include:
● Alcohol dependence.
● Elderly.
● Infants.
● Anticoagulants.
● Idiopathic (5%).

Clinical presentation

These fall into 2 distinct types:
● Acute: these usually present with a headache and a decreasing level of consciousness. There is usually a good preceding history of trauma.
● Chronic: these are more insidious in nature and can develop over weeks. The initial injury may be relatively minor. As these develop over a long timescale this means that there is a far greater opportunity to successfully treat these once diagnosed.

Imaging (Fig. 10.3)

NCCT is the investigation of choice due to its availability. Blood is usually seen in a crescentic configuration adjacent to the skull. Unlike SAHs the blood isn't restricted by the suture lines and can extend over a full hemi-sphere.

Chronic bleeds can be more problematical in that the blood can be the same density as the brain. This can make identification of these very difficult.

MRI is more sensitive than CT at delineating the extent of chronic subdural haematomas as well as underlying brain tissue injury. In addition MRI is far more sensitive at identifying small and isodense haematomas.

Information for the radiologist

The patient's clinical condition and GCS are important. Anaesthetic support may be required.

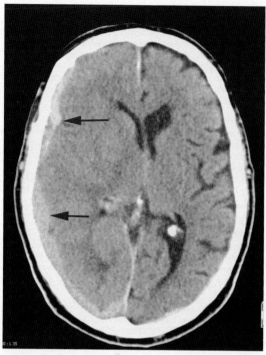

Fig. 10.3 Axial CT head image of a patient with steadily deteriorating gait over the past week and sudden onset of headache 4 hours ago. The 2 arrows point to subdural haemorrhage. The anterior bleed is bright consistent with an acute bleed and the posterior bleed is isodense with the adjacent brain tissue consistent with a 1-week-old bleed. Notice also the ventricular effacement on the right and loss of the grey-white differentiation consistent with raised intracranial pressure.

Encephalitis

Encephalitis is defined as inflammation of the brain parenchyma. It is usually secondary to viral infection, but can also develop secondary to bacterial and fungal meningitis. The most common cause of fatal encephalitis in the UK is herpes simplex virus (HSV-1).

HSV-2 causes congenital encephalitis in neonates. Acute disseminated encephalomyelitis (ADEM) is an immune response to viral infection or less commonly vaccination. It is more common in children.

Clinical presentation

Many encephalitides are mild and self-limiting. Only a minority will develop into a serious illness. Headaches, fever, mood changes, and drowsiness are initial presenting signs and symptoms. Focal neurological signs, seizures, coma, and death or lasting brain injury follow.

ADEM is clinically similar to viral encephalitis, but usually recovers within 2–3 weeks, although 10–20% of patients suffer long-term brain damage.

Imaging

CT (Fig. 10.4)

Subtle oedema, in the temporal lobes and adjacent posterior frontal regions with local mass effect can be seen on NCCT in the first 2–3 days.

These minimal changes are in contrast to marked clinical impairment. Haemorrhage may give rise to areas of patchy increased density. Enhancement following IV contrast is common.

MRI

Gyral oedema is seen as low signal (dark) on T1- and high signal (bright) on T2-weighted and FLAIR sequences. MRI is more sensitive to white matter changes than CT and will demonstrate them both earlier and their full extent. Haemorrhage may be visible as high signal on T1 and signal voids on T2* imaging—these changes imply necrosis. Enhancement following IV gadolinium will be similar to that seen on CT.

Information for the radiologist

The clinical condition of the patient is important. As stated earlier, CT changes may be minimal in a seriously ill patient and may warrant an early MRI. If the patient has a depressed level of consciousness anaesthetic support may be required, see 📖 OHCM, pp. 400 and 834.

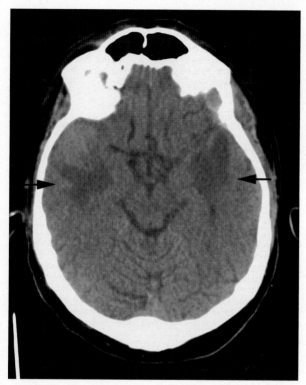

Fig. 10.4 Axial CT image showing low attenuation areas on both temporal lobes (arrows) consistent with herpes simplex encephalitis.

Brain abscess

Brain abscess is a focal infection (usually bacterial) that behaves like an expanding mass. Typical causes are *Streptococcus milleri*, *Bacteroides*, *Staphylococcus*, tuberculosis, fungal, or parasitic infection. Multiple abscesses are seen in immunocompromised patients such as those with HIV/AIDS or following organ transplant. Intravenous drug users (IVDU) are at increased risk.

Clinical presentation

- Headache and focal signs, depending on the location of the abscess are typical.
- Seizures and signs of raised intracranial pressure such as vomiting are common.
- Fever and elevated white cell count, CRP, and ESR are usual.

The duration of clinical symptoms is variable, but cerebellar abscesses may progress rapidly due to hydrocephalus.

Imaging

CT

NCCT will demonstrate low-density area/s. These typically show ring enhancement following IV contrast (Fig. 10.5). The enhancement is due to the breakdown of the blood–brain barrier in the abscess capsule. Other features include surrounding vasogenic oedema (low density) and mass effect such as sulcal effacement and shift of the midline structures.

Hydrocephalus can be seen in association with posterior fossa abscesses. Enhancement of the ventricular lining (ventriculitis) implies intraventricular extension of the abscess, which carries a poorer prognosis.

MRI

On MRI the necrotic abscess centre and surrounding brain oedema will appear hyperintense (bright), similar to CSF, on T2-weighted and FLAIR imaging. The abscess capsule enhances following IV gadolinium on T1-weighted imaging.

Information for the radiologist

Neurological status and GCS will help the radiologist to prioritize investigations. Patients with decreased levels of consciousness, seizures, or focal neurological deficits require urgent imaging. Patients with depressed consciousness may require anaesthetic support.

Further information such as whether the patient is immunocompromised or an IVDU is very helpful.

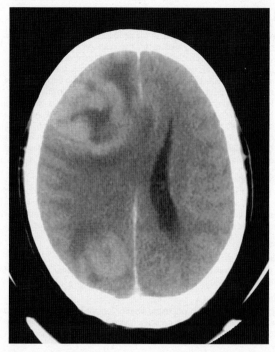

Fig. 10.5 Axial CT showing multiple ring-enhancing lesions within the brain, with significant amount of perilesional oedema, and midline shift in a patient with multifocal abscesses.

Hydrocephalus

Hydrocephalus is an imbalance in the production, flow, and absorption of cerebrospinal fluid (CSF) leading to a rise in interventricular pressure.

- Communicating hydrocephalus occurs when there is either over production of CSF, defective absorption, or venous drainage insufficiency, but there remains open communication between the ventricles and subarachnoid space, e.g. following meningitis or SAH.
- Non-communicating hydrocephalus occurs when there is obstruction to CSF flow either between the ventricles or between the ventricular outflow and the subarachnoid space. This is most commonly caused by either a congenital abnormality or by an intracranial tumour. Stenosis of the aqueduct of Sylvius connecting the 3rd and 4th ventricles is the most common site of congenital obstruction.

Clinical presentation

In adults the most common presentation is of cognitive decline. Other symptoms include headache that is often worst in the morning, nausea, vomiting, and visual disturbance. In children symptoms may be non-specific and include irritability, drowsiness, poor feeding, and headaches.

Imaging

Plain film

In babies and infants there will be bulging of the anterior fontanelle, and widening of the sutures.

Ultrasound

May be used in infants in whom the anterior fontanelle is still patent to assess the size of the ventricles. It is particularly useful in assessing for subependymal and intraventricular haemorrhage, which may lead to hydrocephalus.

CT

There will be enlargement of the ventricles, with rounding of the frontal horn shape and corresponding dilatation of the temporal horns with the lateral ventricles (Fig. 10.6). There will often be periventricular low-density indicating transependymal flow of CSF.

The most important distinction to make is between hydrocephalus and white matter atrophy. Previous imaging may be very useful in making this distinction.

MRI

The same criteria are used for diagnosing hydrocephalus on MR as on CT. Transependymal CSF flow is best appreciated as high signal on FLAIR sequences.

Information for the radiologist

Any previous imaging of the brain is crucial in interpreting the presence or progression of hydrocephalus.

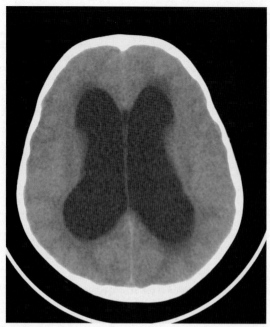

Fig. 10.6 Axial non-contrast-enhanced CT image showing gross dilatation of the ventricles. In addition there is effacement of the sulci. These findings are consistent with hydrocephalus.

Acoustic neuroma

Otherwise known as a vestibular schwannoma. This is a benign intracranial, extra-axial tumour, which arises from the myelin cells of the vestibulocochlear nerve (CN VIII). In 85% they arise from the vestibular portion and in 15% from the cochlear portion. The most common location is the internal auditory canal but they may also arise at the cerebellopontine angle.

Associations

Acoustic neuromas may occur sporadically or as part of von Recklinghausen's neurofibromatosis.

- In neurofibromatosis type I a schwannoma may sporadically involve the VIIIth nerve. Bilateral acoustic neuromas are rare.
- In neurofibromatosis type II bilateral acoustic neuromas are almost pathognomonic. They tend to present below the age of 21.

Clinical presentation

There is usually a long, progressive history of sensorineural hearing loss and most patients also complain of tinnitus. Other symptoms include pain, vertigo, and ataxia. Larger tumours may start to cause symptoms associated with raised intracranial pressure such as nausea, vomiting, headache, and eventually a decreased conscious level.

Imaging

Plain film

There may rarely be erosion of the internal auditory canal.

CT

These usually present as an isodense tumour, on non-enhanced CT, which enhances uniformly following IV contrast. There is no internal calcification within the tumour. CT will detect almost all tumours >2cm in size but it is not so sensitive for very small lesions.

MRI

They are usually darker than brain tissue on T1 and show intense enhancement following IV gadolinium (Fig. 10.7). On T2 imaging the tumour will appear bright.

Angiography

The vascular supply is usually from the external carotid artery. Displacement of the nearby vessels is the most common finding at angiography.

Information for the radiologist

- Does the patient have any other stigmata of neurofibromatosis, e.g. multiple neuromas, café au lait spots, or axillary freckling?
- Are the symptoms unilateral or bilateral?

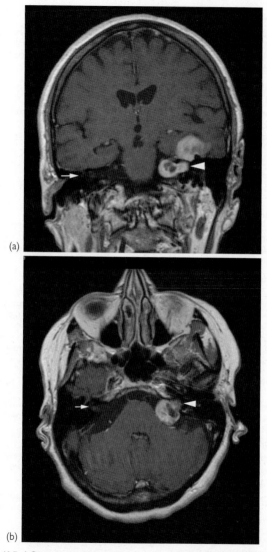

Fig. 10.7 a) Coronal image. b) Axial image, both are T1-weighted post-gadolinium images. The arrow shows the normal right vestibulocochlear nerve with no evidence of enhancement. The arrowhead shows the abnormal nerve on the other side with marked enlargement and significant enhancement.

Glioma

Glioma describes a tumour, which arises from the glial cells. The most common location is the brain, but they also occur in the brainstem, the spinal cord, and the optic nerve. The tumours are further classified according to cell of origin, location, and by grade.

Classification

Cell of origin

- Astrocyte: astrocytoma. Glioblastoma multiforme is the most common type of astrocytoma. These are very aggressive.
- Ependyma: ependymoma.
- Oligodendrocyte: oligodendroglioma.
- Medulloblast: medulloblastoma.

Location

Gliomas may be supratentorial or infratentorial. In adults they are mostly supratentorial and in children mostly infratentorial.

Grade

- Low grade: these tend to be slow growing benign and carry a better prognosis.
- High grade: tend to be more aggressive, malignant, and carry a worse prognosis.

Clinical presentation

This will depend upon the area affected. Brain gliomas cause signs and symptoms associated with raised intracranial pressure such as headache, nausea, vomiting, decreased conscious level, as well as seizures and cranial nerve palsies. Generalized symptoms such as memory loss and personality change are also common.

A glioma originating in the spinal cord may manifest with weakness and paraesthesia in the limbs or with pain in the spine.

Imaging

CT

On NCCT gliomas appears as an irregular and poorly defined low-density area causing mass effect. There will usually be enhancement following IV contrast but the pattern is variable and non-specific.

MRI (Fig. 10.8)

Tumours are typically low signal on T1 imaging and high signal on T2 imaging, usually with surrounding oedema. They enhance following gadolinium.

Angiography

Whilst this technique is unlikely to be used for diagnostic purposes, it may be performed prior to surgical intervention and will often show an extremely irregular vascular pattern.

Information for the radiologist

- Focal neurological signs.
- Are there any signs of cord compression or raised intracranial pressure?

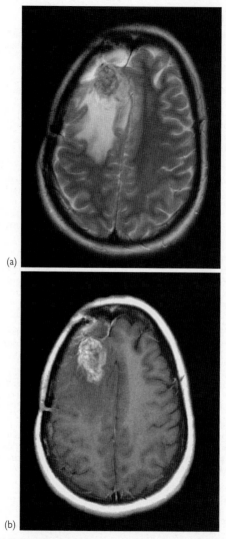

Fig. 10.8 A 25-year-old patient was referred for MRI as they had severe intractable headache with vomiting. a) T2W axial image which shows extensive oedema with a more complex central abnormality in the right. b) T1W Gd axial image showing marked enhancement of the lesion. This was proven to be an astrocytoma.

Meningioma

This is the most common extra-axial tumour in adults. Although usually a benign tumour it can, rarely, undergo malignant transformation. It arises from the meninges and is usually supratentorial in location (90%). They are usually slow growing but may be surgically resected if causing significant symptoms.

The peak age incidence is 45 years and they are relatively rare in children.

There is no known cause but risk factors include:
- Neurofibromatosis type 2.
- Radiation to the head and neck.
- Exposure to female hormones and breast cancer.

Clinical presentation

Symptoms are caused either by direct pressure on underlying brain parenchyma, raised intracranial pressure, involvement of cranial nerves, or involvement of surrounding bone and soft tissues. These include non-specific headaches, seizures, focal weakness, and cranial nerve palsies. However, many are asymptomatic and are purely incidental findings.

Imaging

Plain film

The most common finding on a plain radiograph would be hyperostosis of the bone adjacent to the meningioma. Calcification within the tumour may also be identified.

CT

Usually a well-circumscribed hyperdense, mass seen on NCCT, that has a broad based attachment to the dura. They enhance intensely following IV contrast. There is often internal calcification and hyperostosis of the adjacent bone.

MRI (Fig. 10.9)

On T1 images the lesion will be either low signal or isointense and on T2 will be either isointense or high signal. There is avid contrast enhancement with the administration of gadolinium. Classically a 'dural tail' sign will be seen.

Angiography

Meningiomas are almost always supplied by the external carotid artery and very rarely by the internal carotid artery. A 'mother in law' blush is typical, i.e. contrast shows up early and stays late! There is often a sunburst appearance of the feeding vessels.

Information for the radiologist

- Previous history of radiotherapy.
- Does the patient have neurofibromatosis?

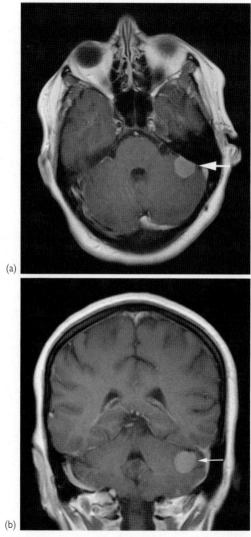

(a)

(b)

Fig. 10.9 a) Axial T1-weighted post gadolinium image. b) Coronal T1-weighted post gadolinium image. The arrows point to a well-defined enhancing lesion attached to the posterior border of the petrous bone consistent with a small meningioma.

Brain metastases

This is one of the most feared complications of systemic cancer by many patients. Metastases are the most common of the intracranial neoplasms and 6 primary tumours account for the majority of all brain metastases. These are: lung, breast, colon, renal, melanoma, and choriocarcinoma.

Clinical presentation

Symptoms are either usually caused by a rise in intracranial pressure with symptoms such as nausea and vomiting, headache, and confusion, or by a focal destruction of neurons at the site of the metastasis producing limb weakness, seizures, visual defects, or speech disturbance. Approximately 2/3 of all brain metastases are symptomatic.

Imaging

Plain film

These are rarely used but lytic or sclerotic lesions on a skull radiograph may be seen if there is bone extension. The most common primary tumours to show this pattern are lung and breast.

CT

In almost all patients presenting with symptoms suggestive of brain metastases CT will be the first investigation. The typical appearance is of low attenuation areas on NCCT, often multiple and usually found at the grey/white matter junction. After IV contrast they will usually enhance and more lesions may become apparent.

MRI (Fig. 10.10)

If there is only one lesion visible on CT then MRI may be used to look for further lesions in order to confirm the diagnosis of metastatic disease. Multiple lesions with surrounding oedema are often seen. These are low signal on T1 and high signal on T2 imaging. Surrounding oedema is usually low signal on T1 and high signal on T2 imaging.

Information for the radiologist

Information about any history or cancer is helpful, even if the cancer was some time ago, it may still be relevant.

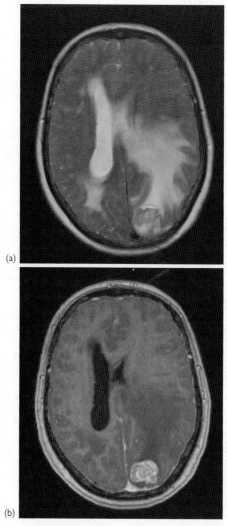

(a)

(b)

Fig. 10.10 A 54-year-old patient with known breast carcinoma with right-sided visual disturbance. a) Axial T2 image with extensive left occipital oedema with a complex lesion, posteriorly. Low-grade oedema on the contralateral side. b) Axial T1 post-gadolinium-enhanced image demonstrating heterogeneous enhancement of the lesion consistent with a metastasis.

Pituitary adenoma

Background

Conditions involving the pituitary gland were first described in 1886 by a French neurologist who studied 2 patients with symptoms suggestive of acromegaly. Pituitary adenomas are benign, slowly growing tumours arising from the anterior lobe of the pituitary gland or adenohypophysis.

Most pituitary adenomas arise spontaneously but can also occur as part of the multiple endocrine neoplasia I (MEN I) syndrome.

Clinical presentation

Symptoms may be due to either a local pressure effect from the tumour itself on surrounding structures, or may be related to distant endocrine manifestations. A large proportion of patients present with visual symptoms due to compression of the optic nerves.

Classification

The tumours are classified according to size: a tumour <10mm is termed a microadenoma and when >10mm is termed a macroadenoma. The functioning tumours are then also classified according to which hormone they secrete.

Prolactinoma

This is the most common of the pituitary adenomas. In women presenting features include amenorrhoea, infertility, and galactorrhoea. In men symptoms include impotence, low libido, and visual disturbance.

Corticotrophic adenoma

This is an ACTH-secreting tumour which causes Cushing's disease—symptoms in this case include weight gain, osteoporosis, muscle weakness, a 'buffalo-hump' at the back of the neck, dryness and thinning of the skin.

Somatotrophic adenoma

These tumours secrete growth hormone causing gigantism in children and acromegaly in adults.

Gonadotropic cell adenoma

These tumours are quite rare and secrete luteinizing hormone and follicle-stimulating hormone. Symptoms in this case include amenorrhoea and impotence.

Thyrotrophic cell adenoma

This tumour secretes thyroid-stimulating hormone and produces signs and symptoms of thyrotoxicosis, such as heat intolerance, sweating, tachycardia, and weight loss. This type of adenoma is often large and invasive.

Imaging

Plain film

Skull radiographs are now relatively rare but occasionally signs of a pituitary adenoma such as enlargement of the sella and erosion of the clinoid processes may be seen. These findings are however non-specific and unreliable!

CT

Microadenomas will usually be seen as a focal hypodensity seen on both non-contrast and contrast-enhanced CT. The adenoma may enhance but not as quickly as the surrounding normal pituitary tissue. Other findings include deviation of the pituitary stalk and erosion of the sella floor.

Macroadenomas have variable appearances but most are isoattenuating relative to the cortex on non-enhanced CT scans and show moderate enhancement on enhanced scans.

MRI (Fig. 10.11)

Coronal T1 images are the most sensitive. Adenomas are usually seen as a focus of low signal on T1 images and a focus of high signal on T2 images.

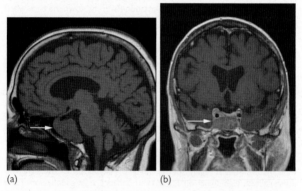

(a)   (b)

Fig. 10.11 a) Sagittal T1-weighted MRI image demonstrating tumour in the pituitary fossa. b) Post-gadolinium enhanced coronal image shows uniform enhancement throughout. This proved to be a prolactinoma.

Multiple sclerosis

This is a demyelinating disease affecting the spinal cord and the brain. The characteristic lesions are called plaques. Multiple sclerosis (MS) usually affects young adults and is more common in females. There is no known definite cause for this and at the present time no curative treatment is available.

Clinical presentation

Due to the nature of the condition it can present with almost any neurological sign or symptom and may progress to cognitive and physical disabilities. The diagnosis requires objective evidence of lesions disseminated in time and space (McDonald criteria[1]). Lhermitte's sign is characteristic but not specific to MS. This is an electrical sensation that runs down the back when bending the neck.

Imaging

Currently a combination of clinical, laboratory, and radiological tests are used to make the diagnosis. The only radiological investigation of routine value is MRI.

MRI (Fig. 10.12)

This is the investigation of choice as no other modality can demonstrate the plaques. A combination of T1-weighted, FLAIR, and post-contrast (gadolinium) enhanced can be used to detect these. The whole of the brain and the spinal cord should be covered.

Classically plaques are seen in the corpus callosum, U-fibres, temporal lobes, brainstem, cerebellum, and the spinal cord. Temporal lobe involvement is highly specific for MS. Plaques show low signal on T1-weighted, high signal on FLAIR, and enhance post-gadolinium in the brain (after they have been present for a month). Dawson's fingers are typical for MS—these are ovoid lesions running perpendicular to the ventricles secondary to inflammation around penetrating venules.

Information for the radiologist

- Has the patient had any other neurological events?
- What is their current neurological status?

Reference

1 McDonald WI, Compston A, Edan G, *et al.* Recommended diagnostic criteria for multiple sclerosis: guidelines from the International Panel on the diagnosis of multiple sclerosis. *Ann Neurol* 2001; **50**(1): 121–7.

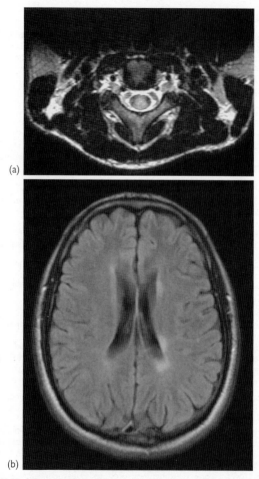

Fig. 10.12 a) T2-weighted axial MRI image from the upper cervical spine showing oedema of the cord consistent with a plaque. b) Axial FLAIR image of the brain. This shows multiple periventricular plaques.

Epilepsy

Epilepsy is a common chronic neurological disorder characterized by the occurrence of at least 2 unprovoked seizures 24 hours apart. Seizures result from an abnormal paroxysmal discharge of cerebral cortical neurons.

Classification

- Generalized seizures:
  - Tonic–clonic (grand mal).
  - Absence (petit mal).
  - Myoclonic (rare involuntary muscle jerks).
- Partial seizures:
  - Simple partial (no impairment of consciousness, e.g. Jacksonian seizures).
  - Complex partial (with impairment of consciousness, e.g. temporal lobe epilepsy).

Clinical presentation

This depends on the location of seizure activity in the cortex as well as the extent and pattern of its propagation in the brain.

Imaging

Neuroimaging should not be routinely requested when a diagnosis of idiopathic generalized epilepsy has been made clinically.

CT

This can be used to identify gross pathology if MRI is not available or is contraindicated.

MRI

This is the imaging investigation of choice in individuals with epilepsy, particularly in those:

- Who develop epilepsy before the age of 2 years or in adulthood.
- Who have any suggestion of a focal onset on history, examination or electroencephalography (EEG).
- In whom seizures continue in spite of first-line medication.

Routine brain MRI may well reveal an underlying cause, such as neoplasia. This should be performed within 4 weeks of presentation (NICE epilepsy guidelines[1]).

The principal role of MRI in epilepsy however, is in the definition of structural abnormalities that underlie seizure activity. In patients with drug-resistant epilepsy, excision of such a lesion may be curative or may improve seizure control.

MR spectroscopy is sometimes used to assess concentrations of cerebral metabolites and some neurotransmitters non-invasively.

Scintigraphy

This can be used as a further means of imaging in potentially preoperative MRI-negative cases. PET may provide data on regional cerebral blood flow, glucose metabolism, and the binding of specific ligands to receptors.

Information for the radiologist

- Symptoms and signs at presentation and current seizure activity.
- Response to medical treatment.
- If surgery is being considered.

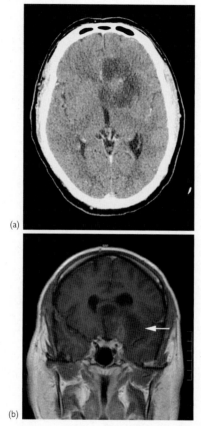

Fig. 10.13 A 30-year-old patient who presented with 3 seizures over a week. a) Axial contrast-enhance CT demonstrating a mixed attenuation lesion anterior left insula region. b) Coronal T1 post gadolinium image confirming this high-grade tumour with extensive oedema.

Reference

1 NICE. The epilepsies: the diagnosis and management of the epilepsies in adults and children in primary and secondary care. London: NICE, 2004.

Head and neck differential diagnosis

Bare orbit

- Neurofibromatosis.
- Metastatic disease.
- Meningioma.

Orbital calcification

- Cataract.
- Retinoblastoma.
- Previous infection.
- Meningioma.
- Vascular calcification.

Absent or hypoplastic paranasal sinuses

- Congenital.
- Down's syndrome.
- Kartagener's syndrome.
- Paget's disease.
- Fibrous dysplasia.

Opacification of maxillary antrum

- Trauma.
- Infection.
- Malignancy.
- Fibrous dysplasia.
- Wegener's granulomatosis.
- Dentigerous/mucous retention cyst.

Nasopharyngeal mass

- Normal adenoids (esp. in children).
- Mass lesions:
  - Nasopharyngeal cancer.
  - Lymphoma.
  - Angiofibroma.
  - Rhabdomyosarcoma.
  - Trauma.
  - Infection.

Head and neck presenting syndromes

Neck lumps

Differential depends on position:
- Superficial (within skin):
  - Lipoma.
  - Sebaceous cyst.
- Anterior triangle:
  - Lymph nodes (reactive or malignant).
  - Branchial cleft cyst.
  - Carotid body tumour.
  - Aneurysm.
  - Vascular malformation.
- Midline:
  - Thyroid mass.
  - Thyroglossal duct cyst.
  - Laryngocoele.
  - Dermoid cyst.
- Submandibular:
  - Lymph node.
  - Salivary gland infection.
  - Salivary gland tumour.
  - Sialolithiasis.
- Posterior triangle:
  - Commonly lymph nodes.
  - Cervical rib.
  - Pharyngeal pouch (rare).

Imaging

Ultrasound
Usual first-line modality for assessment of palpable lumps, it allows accurate localization and characterization, as well as guiding biopsy if required.

CT
Useful in assessment of deeper structures, especially if infection and abscess formation are being considered.

MRI
Gives better soft tissue characterization than CT and should be used if suspecting metastatic disease from a nasopharyngeal and oropharyngeal primary.

Fluoroscopy
Sialography (contrast injection in the salivary gland ducts) gives accurate images of the glandular structure, as well as stones or strictures in the duct.

Nuclear medicine
PET-CT is used in the assessment of malignant lymph nodes with no known primary. Scintigraphy is also used in cases of thyroid and parathyroid enlargement.

Hoarse voice

The commonest causes of a sudden change in voice quality are infection, laryngitis, pharyngitis, and epiglottitis.

Imaging plays a role in cases where direct inspection raises the possibility of tumours on the vocal cord, or recurrent laryngeal nerve palsy.

The left recurrent laryngeal nerve passes into the mediastinum and loops under the aortic arch before coming back up into the neck, and so is potentially involved in diseases affecting the left side of the mediastinum. The right recurrent laryngeal nerve doesn't come so far down, looping under the brachiocephalic artery, and so is less often affected.

Imaging

Plain film

CXR may show a lung or mediastinal mass to account for a laryngeal nerve palsy.

Ultrasound

Little role, but can be used to search for and characterize lymph nodes if appropriate.

CT

Used to stage laryngeal tumours, and to investigate the course of the laryngeal nerve, if vocal cord palsy has been diagnosed at endoscopy.

Dysphagia

Defined as difficulty swallowing, and may be due to problems in the pharynx or lower down in the oesophagus. Pharyngeal causes are often associated with odynophagia (painful swallowing).

Remember gradually progressive dysphagia over several weeks, especially in the elderly, is strongly suggestive of malignancy.

Differential includes:

- Infection:
  - Tonsillitis.
  - Pharyngeal abscess (quinsy).
  - Oesophagitis.
- Foreign body.
- Pharyngeal pouch.
- Malignancy:
  - Pharyngeal.
  - Oesophageal.
  - Gastric.
- Benign oesophageal stricture.
- Globus hystericus.

Imaging

Plain film

Lateral soft tissue view of the neck may reveal a foreign body (if radio-opaque such as a chicken bone) or widening of the pervertebral space in cases of pharyngeal abscess.

CXR will show oesophageal dilatation if significant, or possibly a hiatus hernia.

Fluoroscopy

Contrast swallow studies are used to assess the swallowing mechanism, as well as the structure of the pharynx and oesophagus. Can also demonstrate aspiration and reflux.

CT

To assess the neck and mediastinal structures, especially in cases of extrinsic compression.

MRI

Used to assess pharyngeal malignancy.

Nuclear medicine

PET-CT has an increasing role in the staging of many tumours, including oesophageal.

Head and neck conditions

Nasopharyngeal tumours

Most nasopharyngeal malignancies are squamous cell cancers and they most commonly occur in the lateral wall of nasopharynx within the fossa of Rosenmüller (area around the ostium of Eustachian tube). Men are more frequently affected than women. Risk factors include Epstein–Barr virus, exposure to smoke or to chemical pollutants, and ingestion of salted fish.

Imaging has an important role in staging as well as planning the treatment of nasopharyngeal cancers.

Clinical presentation

The most common presenting symptom is a neck mass due to metastatic lymphadenopathy. Other symptoms include epistaxis, nasal obstruction, hearing loss due to blockage of Eustachian tube, and cranial nerve palsies due to skull base invasion.

T-staging

- Tis: carcinoma *in situ*.
- T1: tumour confined to nasopharynx.
- T2: tumour extends to oropharynx and/or nasal fossa:
  - T2a: without parapharyngeal extension.
  - T2b: with parapharyngeal extension.
- T3: tumour invades bony structures and/or paranasal sinuses.
- T4: tumour with intracranial extension and/or involvement of cranial nerves, infratemporal fossa, hypopharynx, orbit, or masticator space.

Imaging

MRI

The preferred imaging modality for the evaluation of the primary tumour due to better soft tissue contrast and multiplanar capability compared to other modalities (Fig. 13.1).

Ultrasound

Cannot accurately assess the primary tumour but is useful in the assessment of cervical nodal disease, and can also guide biopsy of suspicious lymph nodes.

CT

Useful in the evaluation of nodal involvement. The primary draining lymph nodes from nasopharyngeal cancer are the retropharyngeal nodes. CT also detects early bony cortical invasion.

Nuclear medicine

- PET-CT is used in the assessment of residual and recurrent disease following treatment, looking for metastases, and searching for primary lesions in cases of unexplained nodal disease.
- Biopsy is the only definite way to establish the diagnosis.

Information for the radiologist

- Detailed clinical history and result of endoscopy if already performed.

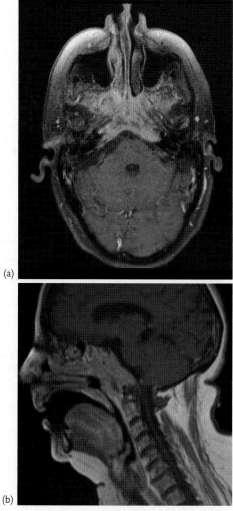

(a)

(b)

Fig. 13.1 a) Axial MR image with gadolinium enhancement revealing a large nasopharyngeal tumour involving the skull base and spreading into the infra temporal fossae on both sides. b) Sagittal MR image of the same patient as (a).

Oropharyngeal tumours

90% of oropharyngeal malignancies are squamous cell cancers. Men are affected three times as frequently as women. Risk factors include heavy smoking, heavy alcohol consumption, chewing tobacco and betel (common in parts of Asia), and human papillomavirus (HPV) infection.

The oropharynx consists of:
- Pharyngeal wall between nasopharynx and pharyngoepiglottic fold.
- Soft palate.
- Tonsils.
- Base of tongue.

Clinical presentation

Patients usually present with dysphagia, persisting sore throat or otalgia but advanced cases may present with trismus or severe pain.

T-staging

- Tis: carcinoma *in situ*.
- T1: tumour ≤2cm in greatest dimension.
- T2: tumour >2cm but ≤4cm in greatest dimension.
- T3: tumour >4cm in greatest dimension.
- T4a: tumour invades any of these: larynx, deep/extrinsic muscle of the tongue, medial pterygoid, hard palate, and mandible.
- T4b: tumour invades any of these: lateral pterygoid muscle, pterygoid plates, lateral nasopharynx, skull base, or encase the carotid artery.

Imaging

Imaging has an important role in defining the extent and accurately staging oropharyngeal tumours. Imaging is also used to monitor response to treatment and can influence treatment choice in certain cases.

Ultrasound

Cannot accurately assess the primary tumour but is useful in the assessment of cervical nodal disease, and can guide biopsy of suspicious lymph nodes.

CT

Useful in evaluating the extent of the primary tumour as well as nodal involvement. It is widely available, has the advantage of speed, and allows chest imaging at the same time (now part of standard staging protocols).

MRI

Superior in the assessment of soft tissue spread, perineural extension, and osseous involvement, particularly if dental amalgam is present (Fig. 13.2).

Nuclear medicine

PET-CT is used in assessing recurrent disease and may have a role in cases of nodal disease with an unknown primary.

Information for the radiologist

Detailed clinical history and result of endoscopy if already performed.

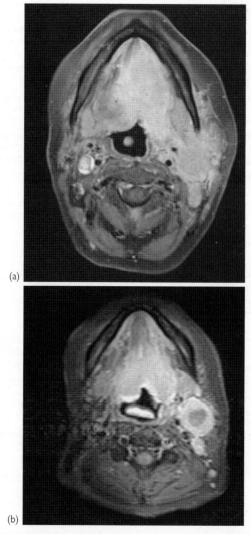

Fig. 13.2 a) Axial MR image revealing a large tumour in the left side of the tongue spreading into the space behind the mandible. b) Gadolinium-enhanced MR image from the same patient as (a) revealing necrosis in the left-sided neck nodes. Biopsy confirmed squamous cell carcinoma.

Laryngeal carcinoma

Carcinomas of the larynx are classified into supraglottic, glottic (true vocal cords) or subglottic depending on the site of origin. 95% are squamous cell carcinomas. Risk factors include smoking and alcohol use.

Glottic carcinoma is the commonest form of laryngeal cancer. It presents early with hoarseness and has the best prognosis.

Supraglottic carcinoma arises above the true cords. Normally presents later, with non-specific symptoms such as dysphagia, odynophagia, and otalgia. Patients may present with a neck mass due to lymphatic spread.

Subglottic carcinoma is the least common. It arises from the undersurface of the vocal cord and usually presents with hoarseness. The subglottis is a difficult area to assess endoscopically and imaging is especially important.

Imaging

Ultrasound
Cannot accurately assess the primary tumour but is useful in the assessment of cervical nodal disease, and can also guide biopsy of suspicious lymph nodes.

CT
The role of imaging is to assess deep and submucosal spread that is blind to the endoscope (Fig. 13.3). CT allows better assessment of the laryngeal cartilages and suffers fewer motion (swallowing and breathing) artefacts than MRI. Regional lymphadenopathy can be assessed and staging is completed with CT of the chest. Coronal reformatted images are useful for assessing the craniocaudal extent of supraglottic tumours and to visualize the superior margin of the true vocal cord.

MRI
Better soft tissue contrast resolution than CT. Useful when cartilage invasion is equivocal on CT, and to assess tumour spread out from the larynx.

Nuclear medicine
PET-CT is used in initial staging and to assess response to therapy.

Information for the radiologist
- Smoking history.
- Endoscopic and clinical findings.
- If recurrence is suspected, details of previous surgery and radiotherapy are very important.

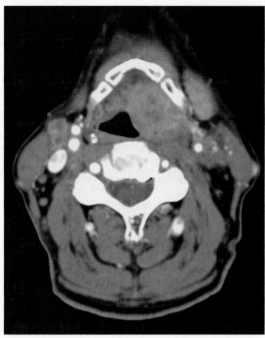

Fig. 13.3 CT image at the level of the hyoid revealing a soft tissue mass in the left side of the larynx with necrotic nodes in the right neck. Biopsy confirmed squamous cell carcinoma.

Thyroid nodules and masses

Thyroid nodules are very common, being found in 4–8% of adults on palpation and in 10–41% by means of ultrasound. The majority are benign, due to cysts, adenomas, or colloid nodules. Although uncommon thyroid cancer may also present as a solitary nodule. Investigation is therefore directed towards discriminating the small percentage of malignant nodules from the large number of benign ones.

Thyroid cancer is classified into papillary (commonest accounting for 60% of cases), follicular, medullary, and anaplastic. Papillary and medullary carcinomas have a high incidence of spread to local lymph nodes whereas follicular carcinoma tends to show early haematogenous spread to lung and bone. Lymphoma and metastases may also present as a thyroid mass.

Presentation

Most patients with thyroid nodules are asymptomatic. A haemorrhagic cyst may present with sudden onset of pain and swelling in the neck.

The presentation of thyroid cancer is variable and depends on the histological type. Neck pain from local invasion, dysphasia, or symptoms of distant metastases can all occur.

Imaging

Plain film

- Limited role but CXR may detect tracheal deviation from retrosternal goitre, mediastinal lymph nodes, and lung metastases.
- Plain radiographs can show metastases in bone, which are usually lytic and expansile.

Ultrasound

The most sensitive method for diagnosing intrathyroid lesions. Features of a benign nodule are a well-defined margin, large cystic component, peripheral 'egg shell' calcification, and lack of internal vascularity.

Features of a malignant lesion include hypoechogenicity, ill-defined margin, fine internal calcification, heterogeneity, and internal vascularity. There is much overlap in these features so fine needle aspiration is often required (Figs. 13.4 and 13.5).

CT

Not sensitive in depicting intrathyroid lesions; however, it is useful for evaluating lymphadenopathy, local tumour extension, and distant metastases from thyroid cancer. It may also be useful for intrathoracic goitre to show its location and extent, to distinguish it from other causes of superior mediastinal mass and assess tracheal compromise.

MRI

Has a limited role in characterizing thyroid nodules, although it is effective in the diagnosis of cervical lymph node metastases and in staging thyroid lymphoma.

Scintigraphy

Used to determine the functional status of nodules. Nodules may be 'cold', 'warm', or 'hot', depending on the uptake of tracer compared with normal thyroid. Thyroid cancers concentrate less radio-iodine than normal thyroid tissue and hence appear 'cold'. Although only 10–25% of cold nodules contain tumour (benign causes include multinodular goitre, focal thyroiditis, and cysts) this finding always requires further assessment.

Technetium-99m pertechnetate is most often used. Gallium-67 scintigraphy is a useful adjunct as thyroid lymphoma is the only thyroid malignancy that takes up this radionuclide.

Information for the radiologist
- The presenting symptoms and signs.
- The results of thyroid function tests.

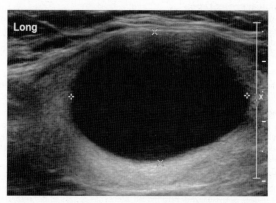

Fig. 13.4 Ultrasound image of the right lobe of thyroid revealing an echo free cyst. There are no features of malignancy and the patient can be reassured.

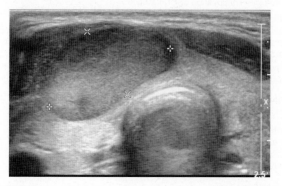

Fig. 13.5 Ultrasound image from a different patient revealing a well defined solid nodule in the thyroid isthmus. Ultrasound-guided fine needle aspiration revealed no malignancy.

Primary hyperparathyroidism

Hyperparathyroidism (HPT) may be primary, secondary, or tertiary. Primary HPT is caused by inappropriate excess of parathyroid hormone (PTH) resulting in hypercalcaemia and hypophosphataemia. It is usually due to a single adenoma, occasionally hyperplasia, and rarely carcinoma. The treatment of a symptomatic parathyroid adenoma is surgical removal. Preoperative localization is the most common indication for imaging of the parathyroid glands. Ectopic glands are seen in 20% of patients and may be found anywhere from the level of the hyoid bone down to the aortic root.

Clinical presentation

Most patients with primary HPT present with mild hypercalcaemia discovered incidentally. More severe hypercalcaemia produces nephrolithiasis, abdominal pain, nausea, constipation, pancreatitis, bone pain, arthralgia, and mental disturbance ('stones, bones, groans, and psychic overtones').

Imaging

Imaging studies should be performed only after the diagnosis of primary HPT is established on the basis of biochemical findings.

Plain film

Radiographs are useful in documenting the effects of HPT upon the bony skeleton, but not the underlying cause. Classic plain film signs include subperiosteal bone resorption on the radial aspects of the phalanges and holes in the bone known as 'Brown's tumours'.

Ultrasound

This is the initial investigation of choice. Normal-sized parathyroid glands are usually not visualized. Parathyroid adenomas appear as discrete, oval, hypoechoic masses, usually posterior to the thyroid gland although their position can be very variable.

Ultrasound-guided fine needle aspiration may be performed to allow cytological confirmation or PTH-assay.

Nuclear medicine (Fig.13.6)

Scintigraphy is the preferred method of examination if ultrasound does not locate the adenoma. Parathyroids and thyroid take up isotopes at different rates and a subtraction method can be used to localize the adenoma.

CT

May be used to detect an ectopic adenoma inaccessible to ultrasound.

MRI

Has better sensitivity than CT for localizing ectopic mediastinal glands.

Information for the radiologist

- Relevant previous surgical history (i.e. of the head/neck/chest).
- Previous or current history of malignancy.
- Any known co-existing thyroid nodules.

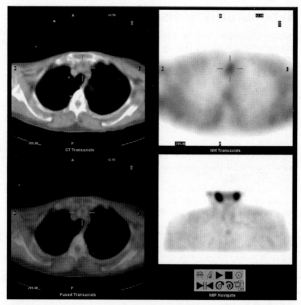

Fig. 13.6 Screen shot images from a SPECT scan showing an ectopic parathyroid adenoma localized to the superior mediastinum. (Image courtesy of Dr Andy Scarsbrook.)

Hypoparathyroidism

Hypoparathyroidism may be congenital or acquired, due to accidental removal of the parathyroid glands during thyroid surgery or their ablation by radio-iodine therapy. Autoimmune disease is a less common cause. Biochemical findings are of hypocalcaemia and hyperphosphataemia.

Clinical presentation

The clinical features of hypoparathyroidism are due to hypocalcaemia. Symptoms include numbness around the mouth and extremities, followed by cramps, tetany (carpopedal spasm), convulsions, and death if untreated.

Imaging

The skeleton is usually normal. The principal radiological manifestation is calcification of the basal ganglia and areas of the cerebrum and cerebellum (seen on CT/MRI).

In pseudohypoparathyroidism (same biochemical findings as hypoparathyroidism but with lack of response to parathormone), affected individuals are short in stature with short metacarpals, metatarsals, and phalanges. The 4th and 5th metacarpals in particular are affected. The teeth are hypoplastic with defective enamel. These changes are best demonstrated on plain radiographs.

Information for the radiologist

Relevant previous surgical history (i.e. of the head/neck/chest).

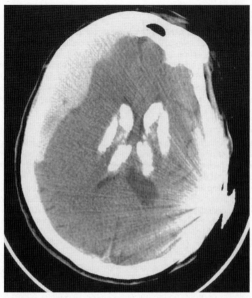

Fig. 13.7 Axial CT showing dense calcification of the basal ganglia due to hypoparathyroidism. There is also an acute right subdural haematoma and artefact from a cochlear implant on the left. Image courtesy of Dr. Daniel Warren.

Sinus disease

Inflammatory sinus disease may be acute or chronic.

Each sinus has its own pattern of mucociliary clearance. Altering normal secretions, ciliary action, or the patency of ostia will result in pathology.

Frontal, anterior ethmoid, and maxillary sinuses all drain into the middle meatus. The region where they drain is the osteomeatal complex (OMC). The sphenoid and posterior ethmoid sinuses drain into the superior meatus. Disease at the OMC causes obstruction of drainage pathways and is a major cause of recurrent acute or chronic sinusitis.

Presentation

Acute sinusitis is often due to secondary bacterial infection following viral upper respiratory tract infection. This results in overproduction of mucus by the inflamed mucosa. Clinically there may be headache, sinus pain, fever, and nasal discharge.

Chronic rhinosinusitis clinically represents recurrent acute sinusitis or a prolonged acute episode refractory to treatment. Other disease entities such as sinonasal polyposis and mucocoeles are often associated with chronic rhinosinusitis.

Imaging

Plain film

Popular historically but are no longer widely used.

CT

The mainstay of modern sinus imaging. Mucosal thickening, polyps, and air fluid levels are all clearly seen, as well as potential complications of acute sinusitis:

- Osteomyelitis: rare with the use of antibiotics.
- Intracranial abscess: spread of infection from the frontal or sphenoid sinuses may give rise to cerebral abscess or subdural empyema.
- Orbital cellulitis: usually follows ethmoid sinusitis and may result in orbital abscess formation.

CT of the sinuses is used in chronic rhinosinusitis prior to functional endoscopic sinus surgery (FESS) to examine the extent of sinus disease, carefully assess the OMC, and note any anatomical variants (Fig. 13.8).

CT can also assess nasal septal deviation and the presence of sinonasal polyposis—which is seen as soft tissue in the nasal cavity, usually arising from the ethmoid sinuses (Fig. 13.9).

MRI

MRI lacks the bony detail of CT but is useful in cases of sinus malignancy.

Information for the radiologist

- Full clinical details including features to suggest a complication of sinusitis.
- Plans for surgery.

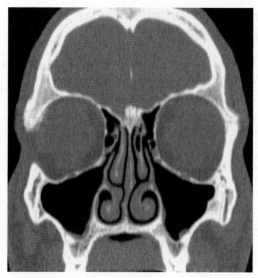

Fig. 13.8 Coronal reformat of a CT through the sinuses, revealing normal anatomy. Note the 2 osteomeatal complexes through which the maxillary sinuses drain into the nose.

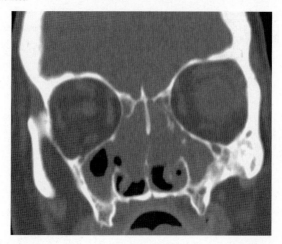

Fig. 13.9 Coronal reformat of a CT revealing extensive nasal and maxillary polyp formation. Note also the previous surgery attempting to improve the sinus drainage by widening the osteomeatal complexes.

Parotid and submandibular salivary glands: infection

Mumps is the commonest cause of acute parotitis but rarely requires imaging. Staphylococcal and streptococcal infections develop in debilitated, dehydrated patients with poor oral hygiene. These patients present with tender swollen glands and systemic signs of infection. Pus may be seen discharging from the parotid duct orifice.

Imaging

Ultrasound
Allows assessment of the gland texture, any underlying duct abnormality, calculi, and abscess formation. Also will demonstrate associated nodes, and allow aspiration if appropriate but it may be difficult to fully assess depth of infection.

CT (Fig. 13.10)
Will show a diffusely swollen gland with inflammatory stranding in the surrounding fat. If an abscess is present this will appear as an area of absent enhancement (dark area within bright gland) or irregular ring enhancement. CT gives a good overall view of the neck and better assessment of deeper structures than ultrasound. Also useful for detecting stones and gas formation.

MRI
Not so good at detecting calculi or gas as CT and little advantage in the acute setting.

Information for the radiologist
- History, especially risk factors such as previous stones, radiotherapy, etc.
- Blood results.

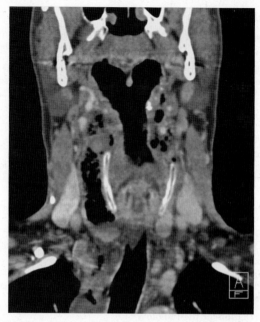

Fig. 13.10 Coronal reformat of a CT from a patient with suppurative infection originating in the salivary glands, now extending throughout the tissue planes of the neck and into the mediastinum.

Sialolithiasis

Salivary gland calculi form as the result of stasis of saliva or infection. They are more common in the submandibular gland (80%) because the saliva is more viscous and the ducts take an uphill course. Patients present with pain and swelling of the affected gland, related to meals. Occasionally the stone may be palpated in the floor of mouth. Sialolithiasis may lead to chronic sclerosing sialadenitis with fibrosis and atrophy of the gland.

Imaging

Plain film

The majority of stones are radio-opaque on plain films.

Ultrasound

Useful initial investigation. Calculi can be identified as an echogenic focus within the gland and associated duct dilatation will also be seen (Fig. 13.11).

CT

Unenhanced scans will demonstrate the stone and then IV contrast can be given to demonstrate any intraglandular abscess.

MRI

Thin section T2 MRI (MR sialography) is less satisfactory for identifying small stones because of signal voids.

Sialography

Contrast injected into the relevant duct opening in the mouth can identify stones and secondary duct dilatation (Fig. 13.12).

Information for the radiologist

Appropriate history and clinical findings.

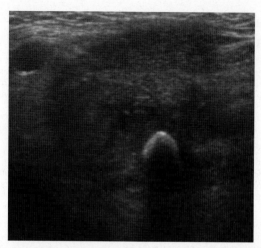

Fig. 13.11 Ultrasound of the submandibular gland reveals a large stone in the duct. Note the dense acoustic shadowing behind it.

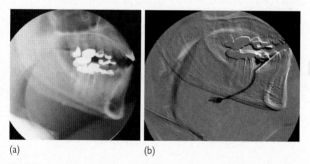

(a)   (b)

Fig. 13.12 a) Control film from a submandibular sialogram reveals a well-defined calculus in the position of the duct. b) Following an injection of iodinated contrast the stone is confirmed to lie within the duct.

Parotid and submandibular salivary glands: tumours

80% of salivary gland tumours arise in the parotid gland. Pleomorphic adenomas are the most common (50%). Patients present with a painless slow growing lump/swelling within the affected gland. Warthin's tumours make up around 10% of benign parotid tumours and are usually found in the parotid tail, occasionally bilaterally.

Carcinomas are less common than benign lesions. Pain, rapid growth, and neurological involvement (facial nerve palsy) all suggest malignancy.

Imaging

Ultrasound

Suspected salivary gland tumours should be investigated by ultrasound in the first instance. Fine needle aspiration can also be performed, but cross-sectional imaging will often be required in addition.

CT

Findings depend on the particular tumour, but in general CT allows easy assessment of all the major salivary glands, tumour extent and depth, and regional nodal involvement (Fig. 13.13).

MRI

Allows more accurate assessment of the facial nerve than CT in cases of parotid malignancy and therefore useful prior to surgery (Fig. 13.14).

Information for the radiologist

- History and clinical findings are important for deciding the most appropriate investigations.
- Contraindications to IV contrast or MRI will help guide imaging.
- If recurrence of malignant disease is suspected then a detailed history of previous surgery and radiotherapy is necessary to interpret difficult imaging findings.

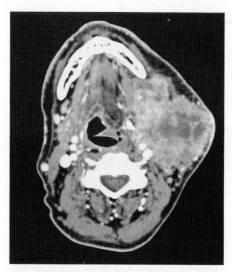

Fig. 13.13 Axial CT image reveals a large, partly necrotic tumour arising from the left parotid. This was a squamous carcinoma.

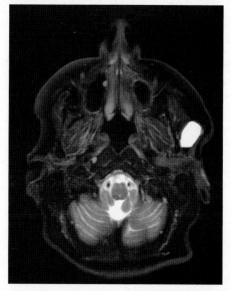

Fig. 13.14 Heavily T2-weighted (with fat saturation) MR image of the left parotid reveals a well defined homogeneous lesion in the gland. Biopsy confirmed a benign cyst.

Branchial cleft cysts

These benign neck cysts usually appear before the age of 30. The 1st branchial cleft develops into the external auditory canal. The 2nd, 3rd, and 4th branchial clefts merge to form the sinus of His, which will normally involute. When a branchial cleft does not properly involute, a branchial cleft cyst forms. See Table 13.1 for classification.

Clinical presentation

Branchial cysts are usually asymptomatic, but they may become painful due to secondary infection. Alternatively, they may present with local mass effect such as respiratory compromise. Fine needle aspiration yields pus-like fluid that is rich in cholesterol crystals. The treatment is surgical excision. However, recurrence rates of up to 20% are reported.

Imaging

Ultrasound

Useful initial investigation of any neck mass (Fig. 13.15a). Although ultrasound can confirm the position and cystic nature of the mass, it does not adequately evaluate the extent and depth of neck lesions.

MRI

This more reliably confirms the cystic nature of the mass and provides precise definition of the extent of the lesion and its relationship to surrounding structures (Fig. 13.15b). MRI is especially advantageous for type I 1st branchial cleft cysts and for parapharyngeal masses that may be 2nd branchial cleft cysts. Wall thickness and enhancement following IV contrast administration varies according to the severity of any associated infective/inflammatory process.

CT

Branchial cleft cysts appear as well-defined, ovoid, fluid-filled lesions.

Information for the radiologist

• Symptoms and signs at presentation.
• Presence of raised inflammatory markers (WCC, CRP).
• Any clinical suspicion of malignancy (metastatic squamous cell carcinoma to cervical nodes may mimic a branchial cleft cyst).

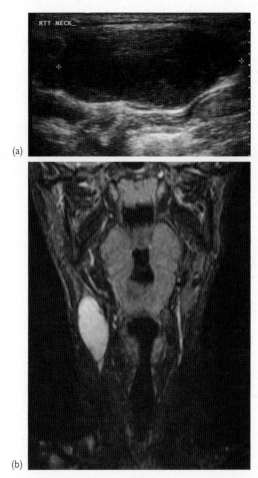

Fig. 13.15 a) Ultrasound image from a 19-year-old man with a painless swelling in the right neck reveals a well-defined cystic lesion. b) Coronal T2c weighted MR scan from the same patient as (a) confirms the anatomical position and benign characteristics of a 2nd branchial cleft cyst.

Table 13.1 Types of branchial cleft cysts

1st	Type I: located near the external auditory canal, most commonly inferior and posterior to the tragus. May also be in the parotid gland or at the angle of the mandible
	Type II: associated with submandibular gland or found in the anterior triangle of the neck
2nd	Accounts for 95% of branchial anomalies
	May present anywhere from the skin of the lateral neck, between the internal and external carotid arteries, and into the palatine tonsil
	Most commonly seen along the anterior border of the upper 1/3 of sternocleidomastoid
3rd	Rare
	Characteristically located deep to sternocleidomastoid within the posterior triangle of the neck
4th	Extremely rare
	Arise in various locations, paralleling the course of the recurrent laryngeal nerve, including the thyroid gland and mediastinum

Genitourinary differential diagnosis

Bladder filling defects

- Blood clot.
- Tumour (transitional cell carcinoma (TCC) adult and rhabdomyosarcoma child).
- Calculus.
- Infection/debris.
- Prostate.
- Foreign body.
- Ureterocoele.

Renal calcification

- Calculi.
- Dystrophic calcification due to localized disease:
  - Infection.
  - Carcinoma.
  - Aneurysm.
- Nephrocalcinosis:
  - Medullary: hyperparathyroidism, renal tubular acidosis, medullary sponge kidney etc.
  - Cortical: acute cortical necrosis, chronic glomerulonephritis, chronic transplant rejection.

Testicular lesions

Testicular masses

- Germ cell tumours (GCTs):
  - Seminoma: most common testicular tumour in adult.
  - Embryonal carcinoma: 20–25% GCT.
  - Choriocarcinoma: rare.
  - Teratoma: 5–10%.
- Non-germ cell tumours: usually benign.
- Lymphoma or leukaemia: may relapse in testis.
- Metastases: kidney, prostate, bronchus, pancreas.
- Orchitis.

Extra testicular masses

- Varicocoele.
- Hydrocoele.
- Hernia.
- Testicular torsion.
- Epididymitis.
- Epididymal cyst.
- Scrotal trauma/oedema.

Causes of hydrocoele

- Congenital.
- Infantile.
- Secondary to trauma, infection, torsion, or neoplasm.

Adrenal calcification

- Cyst.
- Carcinoma: irregular, punctate calcifications.
- Addison's disease.
- Ganglioneuroma.
- Inflammatory: TB/histoplasmosis.
- Phaeochromocytoma.
- Ureterocoele.

Dilated ureter

Obstruction

Within the lumen:
- Calculus.
- Blood clot.
- Sloughed papilla.

In the wall:
- Oedema secondary to a stone.
- Tumour.
- TB.
- Post surgical.
- Ureterocoele.
- Megaureter.

Outside the wall:
- Retroperitoneal fibrosis.
- Carcinoma (cervix, prostate, bladder, rectum).
- Retrocaval ureter.
- Pregnancy/postpartum.

Other:
- VUR.
- Infection.

Genitourinary presenting syndromes

Acute pelvic pain

Acute pelvic pain is a common presenting complaint, especially in women. However, in addition to gynaecological causes there are many other aetiologies:

Causes

Gynaecological
- Ectopic pregnancy.
- Ovarian cyst: haemorrhage, torsion.
- Hydrosalpinx.
- Mittelschmertz.

Urological
- Renal colic.
- Cystitis.
- Acute urinary retention.

Surgical
- Acute appendicitis.
- Diverticulitis.
- Localized perforation.
- Inflammatory bowel disease (although likely to be previous episodes).
- Ruptured iliac aneurysm.
- Strangulated inguinal/femoral hernia.

Clinical presentation

The exact presentation depends on the underlying aetiology.

A thorough history and examination should be conducted in order to establish the most appropriate differential diagnosis.

Symptoms
- Dysuria.
- Frequency.
- Haematuria.
- Signs of sepsis: pyrexia, night sweats.
- Menorrhagia.
- Amenorrhea.
- Increased bowel frequency.

Imaging

Pelvic ultrasound

Transabdominal (TA) ± transvaginal (TV) will aid in diagnosing an ectopic pregnancy or ovarian problems. However, a normal ultrasound in a patient with a positive pregnancy test does not rule out an ectopic.
- Ectopic pregnancy.
- Ovarian cyst ± haemorrhage.
- Dilated fallopian tubes, consistent with hydro-/pyosalpinx.

Renal ultrasound
- Hydronephrosis.
- Urinary calculi.

CT KUB (kidneys, ureters, and bladder)
This is used to look for urinary tract calculi.

CT abdomen and pelvis
- For surgical causes of acute pelvic pain, a CT of the abdomen and pelvis is performed.
- Evaluation of signs of free fluid, gas, and inflammation of the bowel.

Information for the radiologist
- Pregnancy test result.
- Most likely diagnosis—to aid in appropriate imaging choice.
- Creatinine level if IV contrast is to be given.
- Previous history of urinary calculi or tumours.
- History of previous operations.

Chronic pelvic pain

This is a common problem among women aged 20–50 years; accounting for 20–40% of all gynaecological outpatient appointments. The main differential diagnoses include:

- Endometriosis.
- Adenomyosis.
- Pelvic inflammatory disease.
- Pelvic congestion.
- Fibroids.
- Adhesions.
- Irritable bowel syndrome.
- Interstitial cystitis.

Clinical presentation

Considerable overlap of symptoms in these patients:

- Dysmenorrhoea.
- Dyspareunia.
- Menorrhagia.
- Fertility problems.
- Dysuria.

Imaging

Ultrasound: TA ± TV

- Features of endometriosis, e.g. endometrial cysts may be demonstrated. Smaller endometrial deposits are not easily identified on ultrasound.
- Adenomyosis.
- Uterine fibroid.
- Pelvic varices may be demonstrated using Doppler ultrasound.

Pelvic MRI

MR is superior to CT in the investigation of pelvic organs.

- Endometriosis, in particular endometrial deposits, are identified better on MR than using ultrasound.
- Ovarian cysts/masses can be characterized.
- The blood supply to fibroids can be assessed for suitability for embolization techniques.

Hysterosalpingography

This uses a radio-opaque dye to test the patency of the uterine cavity and fallopian tubes.

Venography

This can be used to diagnose and treat pelvic varices in pelvic congestion syndrome.

Angiography

This technique can be used to embolize and therefore cut off the blood supply to treat uterine fibroids.

Acute renal failure

Deterioration in renal function over hours/days, patient is likely to be systemically unwell and is usually oliguric. Determining causation is vital to direct management.

- *Pre-renal cause*: decreased renal perfusion, commonly dehydration. Consider vascular compromise: renal artery stenosis or renal vein thrombosis.
- *Renal cause*: acute tubular necrosis (ATN), glomerulonephritis, or interstitial nephritis. Precipitating factors include circulatory collapse, nephrotoxins, medications, and vasculitis.
- *Post renal cause*: obstructive uropathy. At the renal pelvis or ureteric level the cause may be intraluminal (stones, pus, haematoma), mural (TCC or inflammatory) or extra-mural (intra-abdominal/pelvic malignancy or retroperitoneal fibrosis). Pathology in the bladder or prostate is also a common cause of obstruction. The initial assessment is to measure the urine output with catheterization if required.

Imaging

Ultrasound

To assess for hydronephrosis—if acute this is evidence of obstruction. A cause should be sought such as the presence of a mass or calculi. Renal parenchyma, size and contour of the kidney is important to determine the presence of chronic atrophy.

CT

Caution required for the administration of IV contrast with pre-scan optimal rehydration mandatory. Quoting absolute creatinine levels as a contraindication to IV contrast is a topic for debate and it is probably unhelpful as risk:benefit assessment is required on a case-by-case basis. Post-scan haemofiltration is possible. NCCT scanning is excellent to demonstrate stone disease and upstream obstruction can be observed, replacing the IVU.

Nephrostomy

Percutaneous insertion of a drain through the renal parenchyma into a dilated calyx, with the tip in the renal pelvis. *Indications:* obstructive uropathy to alleviate renal failure and preserve renal function, or to release infection. Septic obstruction or a single functioning obstructed kidney should prompt discussion for on-call intervention.

Information for the radiologist

- Onset of the renal failure, creatinine levels.
- What is the urine output?
- Is there bladder outflow obstruction?
- Lateralizing signs to suggest a kidney or ureteric cause?
- Is there a single functioning kidney?
- Is the patient septic?

Haematuria

Can be frank (visible to inspection) or microscopic (detected on dip test). Always requires investigation which can be done on an urgent outpatient basis if it is the sole presenting feature. Complications can include retention secondary to clots.

Causes
- Suspect bladder and prostate pathology first.
- Stone disease.
- Malignancy (RCC, TCC, prostate).
- Infection.
- Trauma.
- Renal parenchymal disease.
- Urethral pathology.
- March (microtrauma to red cells, seen in runners).
- Haematological paroxysmal nocturnal haemoglobinuria (PNH), bleeding diathesis.

Investigation
- Urine culture and cytology.
- Flexible cystoscopy.
- Renal ultrasound + IVU complete the standard work.
- Retrograde ureterograms/uretroscopy can be performed in theatre by urologists if diagnostic uncertainty remains regarding the upper tracts.
- CT-KUB ± CT-IVU are gaining popularity for the investigation of difficult cases/replacing IVU.

Imaging

Ultrasound
Look for calculi which cast shadows. Assess for renal masses either parenchymal (RCC) or collecting system (TCC). Look for dilatation of the pelvicalyceal system or more focal dilatation of a calyx both of which can indicate obstruction from TCC or stone disease. The bladder should be imaged and a volume obtained post micturition in men to assess for prostatic obstruction. Note ultrasound is no match for cystoscopy in the identification of bladder pathology.

IVU
Declining use as CT urography gains popularity. Contraindicated in renal failure and caution required in patients taking metformin (stop for 48 hours pre test).

CT-KUB/CTU
CT-KUB is a NCCT covering the kidneys, ureters, and bladder and is excellent for demonstrating stone disease. CTU adds a second scan after two boluses of IV contrast 6–8 minutes apart giving excretion and nephrogram phase imaging. It is excellent for demonstrating malignancy.

Hydronephrosis

Dilatation of the renal pelvis, due to urinary tract obstruction. Common causes are:

- Luminal: calculus, blood clot, tumour.
- Wall: ureteric/urethral stricture, congenital bladder neck obstruction/urethral valve, neuropathic bladder.
- Extrinsic: aortic aneurysm, prostatic obstruction, pelvic tumours, diverticulitis.

Clinical presentation

- Loin pain: may be provoked by anything that increases urine volume.
- Complete anuria: suggestive of bilateral obstruction or complete obstruction if single kidney.
- Infection: malaise, fever, and septicaemia.

Imaging

Ultrasound

Once hydronephrosis is established try to find cause:

- Identification of renal or bladder calculi.
- Allows assessment of bladder emptying, therefore signs of bladder outlet obstruction may be identified.
- If a nephrostomy is required (tube in kidney to relieve the obstruction) ultrasound is used to guide the tube into the dilated calyx.

CTU

- Used to look for presence of urinary tract calcification.
- IV contrast is given to assess renal excretion and to look for evidence of any filling defects along the urinary tract (stones or tumours).

MRI

This technique can be used in patients where there is a contraindication to IV contrast.

Nuclear medicine

- Used (more commonly in children) in obstructive uropathies to look at uptake and excretion.
- Differential function is calculated.

Information for the radiologist

- Relevant past medical history, i.e. history of malignancy. Urea and creatinine levels, recent 'trend' in blood results.
- Clotting if an intervention is necessary.

Hypertension

Common medical condition characterized by consistently elevated blood pressure. Defined as >140mmHg systolic or 90mmHg diastolic. Hypertension can be either primary or secondary; primary hypertension essentially means that no cause can be found, accounting for 85–90% of cases. There are many causes of secondary hypertension including chronic renal failure, renal artery stenosis, and tumours such as adrenal adenomas or phaeochromocytomas.

Clinical presentation

Early hypertension is usually asymptomatic but as the condition progresses symptoms include dizziness, nausea and vomiting and visual disturbance. High blood pressure is however a risk factor for many other medical conditions such as stroke, heart attack, aortic aneurysm, cardiac failure and renal failure.

Imaging

Plain film

On a chest X-ray hypertension may manifest with cardiomegaly ± signs of heart failure. In children and young adults coarctation of the aorta may cause hypertension—in this case the classic finding is notching of the inferior surface of the upper ribs.

Ultrasound

Renal ultrasound may be used to look for renal parenchymal disease such as polycystic kidney disease or chronic glomerulonephritis. Renal artery Dopplers can also be measured to assess for signs of renal artery stenosis; however, MRA is more sensitive. Renal tumours such as renal cell carcinoma and Wilms tumour may also rarely cause hypertension.

CT

Tumours causing hypertension, e.g. a phaeochromocytoma, may be picked up on CT. The extent of any atherosclerosis can be assessed, and complications such as aortic aneurysm can be seen.

Angiography

Fibromuscular dysplasia is a cause of renovascular hypertension in the young, particularly women. On angiography the classic finding displayed in the renal arteries is described as the 'string of beads sign'. This represents areas of stenoses interspersed with small aneurysms.

Echocardiography

An echo may show signs of LVH as a result of prolonged systemic hypertension.

Intermenstrual bleeding

Vaginal bleeding (other than postcoital bleeding) which occurs at any time during the menstrual cycle which is not during normal menstruation.

Causes

Many potential causes of intermenstrual bleeding (IMB), some easily diagnosed, others may require imaging. Causes include:

Hormones

- Combined oral contraceptive pill (COCP): either in too low dose or in combination with an enzyme inducing drug.
- Progesterone-only pill.
- Contraceptive depot injections.
- Intrauterine devices.
- Emergency contraception.
- Tamoxifen.

Tumours (benign and malignant)

- Gynaecological cancers including vaginal, cervical, and endometrial cancer.
- Ovarian tumours (usually oestrogen secreting tumours).
- Endometrial and cervical polyps.
- Fibroids.

Others

- Following smear test or treatment to the cervix.
- Caesarean section scars.
- Drugs altering clotting parameters, e.g. anticoagulants, SSRIs, corticosteroids.
- Adenomyosis (ectopic endometrial tissue in the myometrium).

Investigation guidelines

NICE guidelines for patients presenting with IMB are as follows:
- A mandatory full pelvic examination, including cervical speculum examination.
- Do not wait for a smear result or delay due to a previous negative smear result—refer immediately where there is clinical suspicion.
- Consider urgent referral for women with persistent IMB but negative examination findings.

Imaging

Imaging may not be needed in all cases.

Ultrasound

First-line investigation. Usually TA and TV pelvic ultrasound will be performed. The endometrial thickness is measured and images of the ovaries, uterus and adnexae are obtained.

CT

CT is usually a second-line test if ultrasound has been difficult or non-conclusive. It will also be used in staging of cancers such as ovarian cancer.

MRI

Will usually be performed if any abnormality is detected on ultrasound. Pelvic masses are usually characterized using MRI.

Postmenopausal bleeding

Endometrial or vaginal atrophy is the most common cause but more sinister causes such as carcinoma must be ruled out. Other causes include trauma or anticoagulants, hormone replacement therapy, endometrial or cervical polyps, and endometrial hyperplasia.

Imaging

- Gynaecological examination (hysteroscopy) is used in conjunction with imaging.

Ultrasound

TA imaging is performed first to gain images of the pelvis and both kidneys. TV ultrasound is used to measure endometrial thickness, generally the greater the endometrial thickness the greater the chance of sinister pathology. In postmenopausal women, the endometrium should be thinner than in pre-menopausal women. A thickness >5mm is thought to be abnormal. Using this figure of 5mm will mean that sometimes pathology is overlooked, however in cases where clinical suspicion is high then hysteroscopy is also carried out.

CT

CT would not usually be used a first line of investigation. Used in staging of cancers. Intervention such as omental biopsy in cases of ovarian cancer can be performed under CT or ultrasound guidance.

MRI

MRI is useful in characterizing pelvic masses that have been seen on either ultrasound or CT. The MRI characteristics of a mass can be assessed on different sequences to characterize it accurately.

For example, endometrial cancer has slightly lower signal intensity than normal endometrium on T2 imaging; there may also be disruption of the junctional zone.

A definitive diagnosis is of course only made by endometrial biopsy.

Information for the radiologist

Any previous gynaecological surgery should be noted on the request, e.g. hysterectomy and BSO. Any current or previous hormone treatment should also be noted.

Testicular pain

Causes

- Testicular torsion.
- Torsion of the appendix of the testis (hydatid of Morgagni).
- Trauma.
- Testicular tumour (due to haemorrhage within).
- Epididymitis.
- Orchitis.
- Varicocoele.
- Inguinal hernia.
- Segmental testicular infarction.
- Renal colic (radiated pain).

Imaging

Ultrasound

The diagnosis of suspected testicular torsion should be made clinically and investigated by surgical exploration without delay. Only in equivocal cases should imaging be considered (see 📖 Testicular torsion, p. 254 for further details).

Ultrasound using a high-frequency probe is the first-line imaging resource for assessing the scrotum and its contents. It provides high-resolution information of both the testes and related structures. In experienced hands, it can reliably differentiate between the conditions listed earlier and it is cheap, readily available, and quick to perform.

Historically, radionuclide scanning was used in equivocal cases of testicular torsion to assess testicular blood flow. However, it has become a somewhat redundant technique since the advent of ultrasound.

Genitourinary conditions

Bladder and urothelial cancer

- Bladder cancer is the commonest malignancy of the urinary tract; 90% are transitional cell carcinomas (TCCs).
- Risk factors: smoking, aromatic chemical exposure. Other primaries of the renal tract include squamous cell cancer (associated with repeated infection or stone disease) and adenocarcinoma.
- 30% multifocal, usually with additional sites within the bladder although between 1–5% may have proximal disease. Metachronous disease evolves in up to 25% of cases.

Clinical presentation

- Commonly haematuria although UTI, dysuria, pyuria, and flank pain account for a significant number.
- Initial investigations include FBC, U&Es, urine cytology, and cystoscopy.

TNM staging

- Tis: carcinoma *in situ*.
- T1: subepithelial invasion.
- T2: muscularis invasion.
- T3: perivesical invasion.
- T4: invades side wall, adjacent organ or into perinephric fat for renal TCC.
- N0: no node spread.
- N1: single node <2cm.
- N2: single node 2–5cm or multiple small nodes.
- N3: single node >5cm or multiple nodes >2cm.
- M1: distant metastasis.

Imaging

Ultrasound (Fig. 16.1a)

First-line investigation. Echogenic lesions are seen in the bladder lumen, arising from the wall. May see hydronephrosis. Limitations include evaluation of wall invasion and detection of lymph nodes.

CT (Fig. 16.1b)

CT urography used to demonstrate the upper tracts where initial investigations have not demonstrated pathology, as an alternative to the conventional approach of retrograde pyelograms/uretroscopy performed by urologists in theatre. TCC appears as a filling defect in the contrast. CT can assess tumour size, local invasion, and hydronephrosis. Staging CT is performed if malignancy is known, looking for nodal and metastatic disease.

MRI

MRI scan can be used for local staging in the pelvis but not as a routine investigation in most units.

Scintigraphy

Demonstrates areas of increased osteoblastic activity associated with metastatic deposits.

Information for the radiologist
- Presenting symptoms including findings which suggest metastases.
- Biopsy and cytology results.
- Surgical history including previous sites of disease, resections and therapy regimens.
- Renal function if having CT.

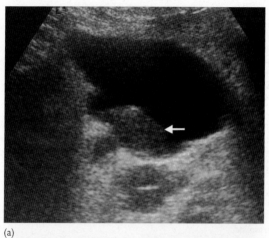

(a)

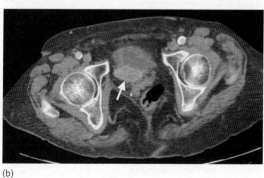

(b)

Fig. 16.1 a) Ultrasound and b) axial CT showing a filling defect within the right side of the bladder (arrows), in a patient with biopsy proven tumour.

Renal cell cancer

- 8th most common malignancy, the peak incidence is in 6th and 7th decades. Male: female = 2:1.
- Associations: long-term dialysis, von Hippel–Lindau syndrome, obesity, smoking, exposure to petroleum products, heavy metals, and asbestos.
- Survival is directly linked to stage at presentation with a >50% 5-year survival for stage II disease and >70% for stage I disease. Metachronous metastases develop in up to 30% predicted by involvement of local lymph nodes. Local recurrence in 5%.

Clinical presentation

- Haematuria, flank pain, and a palpable mass are the classical features; however, only around 10% will have all 3.
- Systemic symptoms include lethargy and weight loss. Calcium and erythropoietin levels should be checked.

Robson's staging system

- I: tumour confined to kidney (large or small).
- II: spread to perinephric fat but within Gerotas fascia.
- IIIA: spread to renal vein or vena cava.
- IIIB: spread to local lymph nodes.
- IIIC: spread to both venous system and local lymph nodes.
- IVA: spread to adjacent organs (excludes ipsilateral adrenal).
- IVB: presence of distant metastases.

Imaging

Ultrasound
Performed as a first-line investigation for haematuria. Excellent detection of renal lesions including solid and cystic masses. Provides Doppler blood flow information regarding invasion of the renal vein or IVC.

CT (Fig. 16.2)
Performed pre- and post-IV contrast for lesion analysis, in particular the presence of enhancement. If a suspected malignant lesion is present a full chest, abdomen/pelvis staging scan should be performed to assess local stage, lymph-nodes, vascular invasion, and metastases.

Bone scintigraphy
Performed to assess for skeletal metastatic disease in the presence of clinical suspicion. Metastases show high tracer activity due to increased osteoblastic activity. Metastases on plain film are typically lucent and expansile.

Information for the radiologist

- Presenting symptoms, relevant medical history and test results including previous imaging.
- Sites of clinically suspected metastases should be highlighted.

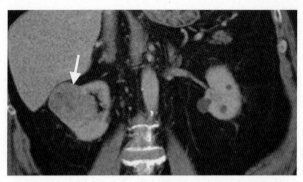

Fig. 16.2 Coronal CT image showing solid mass arising from the right kidney (arrow), renal cell cancer, in contrast to the well-rounded, low attenuation simple cysts in the left kidney.

Testicular cancer

- 95% are germ cell tumours, typical affect men aged 15–45 years. Divided into non-seminomatous (NSGCT) and seminomatous germ cell tumours.
- NSGCT include teratomas, affect a younger age, 10–20 years. Seminomas peak incidence 30–40 years.
- Tumour markers include α-fetoprotein (AFP), hCG (mainly NSGCT), and lactic dehydrogenase (LDH) (both).
- In the UK 1 in 500 men.
- Risk factors: cryptorchidism, genetic predisposition and malignancy in the contralateral testis.
- Treatment is dependent on pathology and stage with NSGCT responding better to chemotherapy and seminomas to radiotherapy.

Clinical presentation

Usually with a hard lump in the testis. Pain and tenderness are less common and usually mild.

TNM staging

- Tis: intratubular neoplasia.
- T1: tumour not invading lymphatics, vessels or tunica vaginalis.
- T2: vascular/lymphatic invasion and/or invasion of tunica vaginalis.
- T3: invades spermatic cord.
- T4: invades scrotum.
- N1: regional nodes (ipsilateral aorto-caval) <2cm greatest dimension.
- N2: regional nodes <5cm greatest dimension.
- N3: regional nodes >5cm greatest dimension.
- M1a: non-regional lymph nodes or pulmonary metastases.
- M1b: other distant metastases.

Imaging

Ultrasound (Fig. 16.3)

First-line investigation. Typically hypoechoic, irregular with increased blood flow.

CT

Used for staging, looking for lymphadenopathy and metastases. Spread is primarily lymphatic to the retroperitoneal aorto-caval nodes, consistent with the embryological origin of the testis. Mediastinal nodes are seen in more advanced disease. Haematological spread is most commonly to the lungs and more rarely to brain, bone, liver, and other abdominal viscera. FDG PET scanning may have a future role in determining residual disease sites to direct the need for further treatment but it is not used routinely at present.

MRI

Not used routinely in the diagnosis or staging of testicular cancer but is useful in detecting cryptorchidism when ultrasound has failed to localize. It offers a wide field of view from mid abdomen through the inguinal canal into the scrotum.

Information for the radiologist
Presence of a lump, relevant past history.

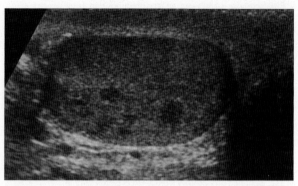

Fig. 16.3 Testicular ultrasound showing multifocal low echogenicity lesion within the testis in a patient with multifocal germ cell tumours.

Prostate cancer

- 2nd leading cause of cancer deaths in males in UK.
- Risk factors: age >50 years, genetic predisposition, familial/racial preponderance Afro-Caribbean >Caucasian >Asian.
- Distinction made between clinical prostate cancer and microscopic, up to 30% men >50 years thought to harbour the disease, most of which will never become apparent.

Clinical presentation

Symptoms of prostatism, haematuria, urinary obstruction, or metastatic disease; however, an increasing number present with an abnormal digital rectal examination (DRE) or an elevated prostate specific antigen (PSA). PSA screening is not performed in the UK at present but has gained popularity in the USA and some of Europe.

TNM staging

- T1a: on histology only from a TURP malignancy in <5% of sample.
- T1b: on histology only from a TURP malignancy in >5% of sample.
- T1c: identified on histology from a TRUS biopsy sample.
- T2a: less than half of one lobe (DRE or imaging).
- T2b: more than half of one lobe (DRE or imaging).
- T2c: involves both lobes (DRE or imaging).
- T3a: extra-capsular extension.
- T3b: extra-capsular extension involves the seminal vesicles.
- T4: invades local structures other than seminal vesicles.
- N1: one or more regional nodes involved.
- M1a: distant (outside the pelvis) lymph nodes involved.
- M1b: bone metastases.
- M1c: non-bone metastases.

Imaging

Plain film and bone scintigraphy

Useful to determine the presence of bone metastases. Often sclerotic on plain film. 'Hot' osteoblastic reaction is seen on bone scanning. Request if symptomatic or PSA markedly elevated.

Ultrasound: trans-rectal ultrasound guided biopsy (TRUS)

The accepted method of obtaining tissue for diagnosis in patients with a raised PSA and suspicion of prostate cancer. Non-targeted 'random' samples are aimed at the peripheral zone of the gland, due to the known preponderance of disease here (>70%).

CT

Staging CT advised if PSA >20, T ≥3, Gleason grade ≥8 or symptoms suggest metastatic spread. Looking for upper tract obstruction, lymphadenopathy, and metastases.

MRI (Fig. 16.4)

Used for local staging to predict spread through the prostatic capsule—important to determine operative or conservative management. It can predict lymph node involvement and bone metastases but is limited by the field of view. Some centres advocate full spinal acquisitions to stage for bone metastases in clinical/biochemically appropriate cases.

Information for the radiologist

PSA level and presence of symptoms suggestive of metastases.

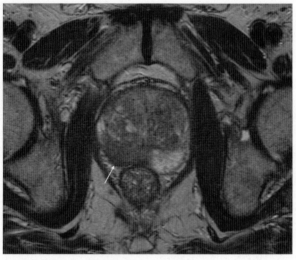

Fig. 16.4 Axial MRI showing a bulky prostate, with a low signal intensity area within the peripheral aspect of the right prostate (arrow). The posterior margin of the prostate is blurred, in keeping with early T3 disease.

Cervical cancer

- 3rd most common malignancy worldwide, average age at diagnosis is 50 years.
- 90% squamous carcinomas, from squamocolumnar junction; 10% adenocarcinomas/adenosquamous carcinomas, arising from glandular elements within the endocervical canal.

Clinical presentation

Vaginal bleeding or discharge. Pain suggests more advanced disease. May be asymptomatic if screen detected.

Staging (see Table 16.1)

Table 16.1 Staging of cervical cancer

FIGO stage	MRI features
0: carcinoma *in situ*	Normal
IA: microscopic invasive	Normal
IB1: clinically visible tumour <4cm	Intermediate signal tumour on T2-weighted imaging replaces dark cervical stroma. An intact stromal ring around tumour indicates tumour confined to cervix
IB2: clinically visible tumour >4cm	
IIA: invasion of tumour to upper 2/3 vagina, no parametrial invasion	Loss of integrity of low signal vaginal wall on T2-weighted sequences
IIB: parametrial invasion but not to pelvic side wall	Dark cervical stromal ring completely replaced by intermediate signal tumour
IIIA: tumour extends to lower 1/3 vagina, not to pelvic side wall	Disruption of the vaginal wall extends to the lower 1/3
IIIB: extension to pelvic side wall or hydronephrosis	Tumour extends to within 1cm of the pelvic side walls or there is ureteric dilatation due to obstruction from the tumour
IVA: bladder or rectal mucosa invaded by tumour	Bladder or rectal wall on T2-weighted images is breached
IVB: distant metastases	Tumour outside the true pelvis

Imaging

Preoperative staging to determine the size and extent of tumour, lymph node status and presence of distant metastases.

Ultrasound

Transrectal ± transvaginal scanning may determine tumour size and extent. The limited field of view reduces assessment of bulky tumours and lymph nodes.

CT

Useful in advanced disease but not accurate in staging early stage tumours. Assessment of local complications, e.g. hydronephrosis, lymphadenopathy, and detection of distant metastases.

MRI (Fig. 16.5)

Most accurate staging method preoperatively, determining tumour size, volume, extent, and nodal status with an overall accuracy of 86–90%. It is also useful to monitor treatment response.

FDG-PET

Main advantage is in detection of lymph node metastases in the pelvis and retroperitoneum. It is also useful in the detection of recurrence of cervical tumour.

Information for the radiologist

Accurate clinical and EUA findings.

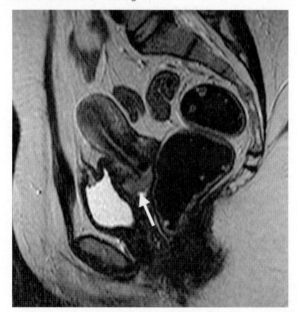

Fig. 16.5 Sagittal MRI showing exophytic tumour (arrow) arising from the cervix, in a patient with a tumour of the cervix.

Endometrial cancer

- One of the most common female pelvic malignancies, usually adenocarcinoma. Less common histological types include serous papillary carcinoma, clear cell carcinoma and undifferentiated carcinoma, which are more aggressive.
- Predominantly occurs in postmenopausal women.
- Risk factors: hypertension, obesity, diabetes mellitus, late menopause, long-term tamoxifen treatment for breast cancer, a personal or family history of breast or ovarian cancer, and a family history of endometrial or breast cancer, hereditary non-polyposis colorectal cancer.

Clinical presentation

Postmenopausal vaginal bleeding or vaginal discharge.

Staging (see Table 16.2)

Table 16.2 Staging of endometrial cancer

FIGO stage	MRI features
IA: confined to endometrium	Junctional zone intact, smooth interface between endometrium and myometrium
IB: <50% invasion into myometrium	Tumour signal extends into superficial myometrium. Irregular interface between endometrium and myometrium
IC: >50% invasion into myometrium	Tumour signal intensity extends into outer half of myometrium. Serosal surface of myometrium maintained
IIA: extension into endocervix	Tumour signal extends into internal os and widens endocervical canal. Cervical stroma intact
IIB: cervical stromal invasion	Dark signal of cervical stroma interrupted by hyperintense tumour signal
IIIA: spread outside uterus into adnexa	Serosal surface disrupted, direct extension into ovaries or discrete ovarian metastases
IIIB: vaginal involvement	Dark T2-weighted signal of vaginal wall invaded by hyperintense tumour
IIIC: lymph node involvement	LN metastases suggested if >1cm in short axis. Also morphological features such as altered signal of LN, irregular margins, extension outside LN capsule
IVA: bladder or rectum involvement	Loss of T2-weighted dark signal of walls of bladder and rectum
IVB	Distant metastases

Imaging

Ultrasound (Fig. 16.6)

TV ultrasound is the first-line test. Look for:

- Endometrial thickness of >4mm: detects 95% of endometrial carcinoma (may be thicker if on hormone replacement therapy/tamoxifen).
- Abnormal endometrium is heterogeneous, hyperechoic, and irregular.

- If there is bleeding, a biopsy is required if the endometrial thickness measures >4mm.
- Endometrial thickness >8mm: with or without bleeding requires biopsy.
- Hysterosonography is a useful adjunct to conventional TV ultrasound, although not widely available. 5ml saline is introduced into the uterine cavity using a catheter, this helps the TV ultrasound to delineate causes such as submucosal myomas or polyps.

CT
May demonstrate pelvic disease and para-aortic lymph node involvement. Not good at local staging.

MRI
Used to locally stage endometrial carcinoma pre-operatively, looking for disruption of normal zonal anatomy and to plan treatment.

Information for the radiologist
Any salient clinical findings and tumour grade and histology if known.

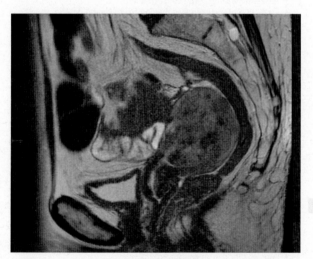

Fig. 16.6 Sagittal T2-weighted image through the midline of the pelvis, showing a bulky mass arising from the endometrium of the upper uterus. This was found to be endometrial adenocarcinoma at histopathology, following hysterectomy.

Ovarian masses

There is a broad spectrum of masses, ranging from physiological cysts to malignant tumours. It is beyond the scope of this chapter to detail every ovarian mass. Instead the broad concepts of imaging and characterization will be described. (See also 📖 Ovarian cancer, p. 230.)

Clinical presentation

Depends on the underlying pathology. Abdominal pain may be a presenting feature if there has been an acute event, such as haemorrhage into a cyst. Ovarian cancer tends to present late with abdominal distention.

Imaging

- Confirm the presence and characteristics of a pelvic mass and determine its organ of origin.
- In cases of malignant tumours, imaging is used for:
  - Preoperative staging.
  - Assessment of response to treatment.
  - Detection of recurrence in the context of clinical deterioration or worsening tumour markers.
  - Guiding percutaneous biopsies/aspiration of ascites.

Ultrasound

First-line investigation. There is much overlap between benign and malignant tumours, although certain features may suggest a particular tumour type. It may be necessary to repeat an ultrasound after a 6-week interval to establish whether the ovarian mass identified is physiological and potentially will resolve.

CT (Fig. 16.7)

May detect incidental ovarian masses, due to the widespread use of this modality. Cysts associated with the ovary that are >3.5cm should be followed up with ultrasound in 6 weeks to ensure resolution.

MRI

Provides excellent tissue contrast and high spatial resolution. MRI may be used if the mass:
- Is large (>10cm).
- Is complex or indeterminate on ultrasound. MRI can accurately determine malignant from benign features, e.g.:
  - Intralesional fat in keeping with a teratoma.
  - Altered blood in an endometrioma.
  - Fibrous tissue, observed in ovarian fibromas or brenners tumours.

Information for the radiologist

History and examination, tumour markers such as CA-125.

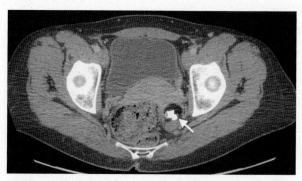

Fig. 16.7 Axial CT showing a mixed attenuation mass within the left adnexa. This contains fat (dark) and calcified teeth (arrow) in keeping with a dermoid tumour.

Ovarian cancer

- 5th leading cause of death from cancer in women.
- >90% epithelial, arising from epithelium ovary/tube. Rarer types include germ cell tumour or sex cord/stromal tumours.
- Risk increases with age and decreases with pregnancy. Associated with *BRCA1* and *BRCA2* gene mutations.

Clinical presentation

Often non-specific symptoms, such as abdominal pain, mass, bloating. Late presentations include leg oedema due to pelvic vein pressures from pelvic mass. Associated with raised CA-125.

Imaging

Ultrasound (Fig. 16.8a)

First-line investigation to assess the ovaries. Ultrasound findings suggestive of a malignant tumour:

- Ovarian cyst >10cm.
- Thick internal septa >3mm.
- Solid component in a cystic mass.
- Colour Doppler flow in the solid elements.
- Presence of ascites.
- Presence of peritoneal nodules.

CT (Fig. 16.8b)

CT features suggestive of a malignant ovarian tumour include:

- The presence of bilateral adnexal masses.
- Mixed solid and cystic components.
- Enhancement of solid components after IV contrast.
- Necrosis in a solid tumour.
- Irregular, thick septae >3mm within a cystic mass.
- Papillary nodules within a cystic mass.
- Presence of lymphadenopathy.
- Invasion into other pelvic organs.
- Ascites.
- Serosal or peritoneal deposits.

MRI

The following MR features are suggestive of malignancy:

- The presence of solid components that have early strong uptake of gadolinium.
- Papillary projections: one of the most significant indicators of malignancy.
- Secondary malignant features such as ascites, invasion of pelvic organs, and enlarged lymph nodes.

Information for the radiologist

History and clinical examination findings, tumour markers.

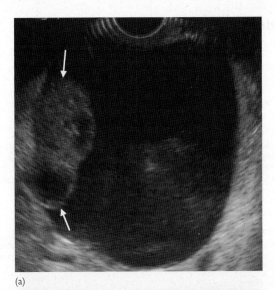

(a)

(b)

Fig. 16.8 a) Ultrasound showing complex ovarian cyst in a patient with raised CA-125. The cyst contains a mural nodule (arrows) and debris. This was an ovarian cancer. b) Axial CT in a patient with bilateral adnexal masses (not shown). The CT shows ascites, and a thick 'cake' of omental disease (arrow). This was due to advanced ovarian cancer.

Adrenal masses

- Common incidental finding ≈1% of abdominal CT exams.
- Non-functioning lesions are benign or malignant. Benign lesions include adenoma, myelolipoma, and haemorrhage. Malignant lesions may be primary or secondary. Functioning adrenal tumours may be:
  - Aldosterone secreting tumour.
  - Phaeochromocytoma.
  - Cushing's syndrome.

Clinical presentation

Majority asymptomatic. Metastatic lesions may be discovered as part of a staging scan. Commonest metastasis to the adrenal glands is from lung cancer followed by breast in women and renal cell carcinoma in men, but even in patients with known cancer, an adrenal lesion found on imaging has only a 26–37% chance of malignancy.[1]

Phaeochromocytoma presents with headache, sweating, flushing, and palpitations, and are bilateral <10% cases.

Imaging

The most important distinction for the radiologist to make is whether the lesion can be considered incidental and benign or whether further investigation is needed.

Plain film

Adrenal calcification is a relatively common phenomenon with causes including: carcinoma, adenoma, neuroblastoma, phaeochromocytoma, infection such as TB or previous haemorrhage.

CT (Fig. 16.9a)

Size is a useful indicator. As a general rule lesions >3cm are more likely to be malignant than those <3cm. Attenuation of the lesion is probably the most useful characteristic. Low attenuation lesions <10HU are usually benign, lesions >10HU are indeterminate. Washout characteristics following IV contrast are also helpful.

MRI (Fig. 16.9b)

MRI is often used to clarify the nature of an adrenal lesion seen on CT. The major distinction is whether or not the lesions contain fat, as this is an indicator of benignity.

PET

A standardized uptake value (SUV) of >4 is indicative of metastatic disease.

Information for the radiologist

Any symptoms or history of malignancy.

Reference

1 Boland GW, Goldberg MA, Lee MJ, *et al.* Indeterminate adrenal mass in patients with cancer: Evaluation at PET with 2-(F-18)-flouro-2 deoxy-D glucose. *Radiology* 1995; **194**:131–4.

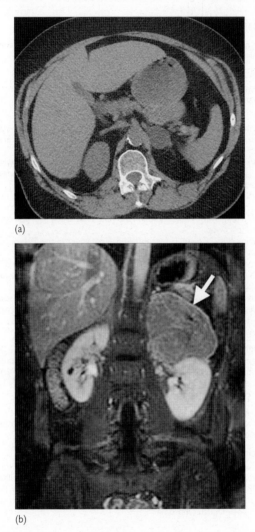

(a)

(b)

Fig. 16.9 a) Non-enhanced axial CT showing fat attenuation nodule within the left adrenal gland, in keeping with a lipid-rich adenoma. b) Coronal MRI showing enhancing, solid mass arising from the left adrenal gland (arrow) found to be a phaeochromocytoma.

Benign renal masses

Often an incidental finding. Role of the radiologist is to decide if the lesion is benign, requires follow-up, or is malignant.

Clinical presentation

Asymptomatic or local symptoms such as flank pain or retroperitoneal haemorrhage.

Cysts

Described using the Bosniak classification system. Class I and II cysts are best imaged with ultrasound, CT is to be used as a problem solver, and MRI to follow-up more complex cases.

- *Bosniak class 1 cysts:* referred to as 'simple cysts': thin wall, near water density. Often multiple, usually of no consequence unless associated with polycystic kidney disease.
- *Bosniak class 2 cysts:* this group contains: non-enhancing hyperdense cysts (haemorrhagic) <3cm, cysts with a single thin septation or cysts with a thin layer of calcification in the wall. They are benign and do not need follow-up.
- *Bosniak class 2F cysts:* 'F' for follow-up. Contain >1 of the features of class 2 cysts or numerous septa, also hyperdense cysts >3cm.
- *Bosniak class 3 cysts:* indeterminate lesions—cysts with evidence of wall thickening, mild nodularity, coarse calcification, septal enhancement. Require consideration for surgical resection.
- *Bosniak class 4 cysts:* cystic carcinoma. Enhancing thick wall with soft tissue components. Enhancement generally considered as an increase in attenuation of >10 Hounsfield (CT density) units after contrast. Managed surgically.

Angiomyolipoma (renal hamartoma)

Contain fat, blood vessels, and connective tissue. If >4cm have increased risk of retroperitoneal haemorrhage. Usually appear bright on ultrasound. Can be safely diagnosed on CT (thin slice) and MR scanning (T1 and opposed phase) by demonstrating fat within the lesion.

Abscess

Can extend into the retroperitoneum. CT gives best demonstration of size and extent.

Imaging

Start with ultrasound, use cross-sectional imaging (CT) as a problem solver (Fig. 16.10). Consider radiation dose if lesions are to be followed up. MRI can help in complex cases and is ideal for following-up patients with multiple lesions at risk of malignant transformation such as in Von-Hippel–Lindau syndrome.

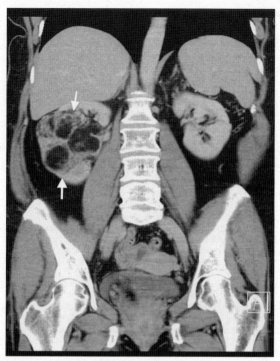

Fig. 16.10 Coronal CT in a patient with right-sided angiomyolipoma (arrows). The CT shows a mass containing fatty (dark) and soft tissue elements (lighter septations). In view of its large size, this was embolized.

Pyelonephrosis

Any condition affecting the renal pelvis; however, often used interchangeably with acute pyelonephritis which is a clinical diagnosis. Chronic pyelonephritis is typically atrophic kidneys following repeated infection/ obstruction, usually related to vesico-ureteric reflux.

- *Acute pyelonephritis*: defined as flank pain, bacteriuria, and pyrexia. 85% caused by ascending UTI. 15% from haematogenous spread. Risk factors include stone disease, diabetes, vesico-ureteric junction reflux, and pregnancy. The role of imaging is to identify obstruction, elucidate causation, and detect complications such as abscess formation.
- *Emphysematous pyelonephritis*: seen with severe infection in diabetics often in an older age group; thankfully rare. There is renal parenchymal gas and destruction, gas can spread in perinephric space and collecting system. NCCT is advised. Prognosis is poor.
- *Renal tuberculosis*: infection via haematogenous route following pulmonary TB, often in immunocompromised. Half will have an abnormal CXR. Presentation is with haematuria, flank pain, sterile pyuria (it is difficult to culture TB, at least 3 samples advised). Pathological changes include destruction of the papilla, strictures, intrarenal cavitations, abscess formation, fistulas, and calcification. Disease progression can descend the ureters into the bladder, prostate, and seminal vesicles however this is rare. Imaging is with CT, CTU or IVU.
- *Xanthogranulomatous pyelonephritis*: chronic inflammatory reaction following repeated infections usually with *Proteus* and is associated with stone disease. Can be focal or diffuse. Imaging demonstrates low density filling of the pelvicalyceal system and ureters.
- *Papillary necrosis*: ischaemic sloughing of the papilla, causes include analgesic NSAID abuse, sickle cell disease, diabetes, and repeated infection. Detached papilla can be seen as filling defects in the collecting system best demonstrated on IVU or CT-IVU.

Imaging

Ultrasound is the initial test to identify obstruction and can show pelvicalyceal pathology/calculi. CT provides extra information regarding causation, extent of disease, and extra renal complications (Fig. 16.11). CT-IVU can assess renal function, pelvicalyceal and ureteric pathologies demonstrated as filling defects within excreted contrast in the collecting systems.

Information for the radiologist

Signs and symptoms and suspected clinical diagnosis.

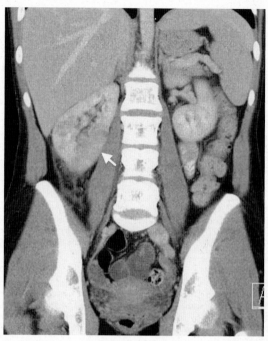

Fig. 16.11 Coronal CT showing ill-defined area of low attenuation (arrow) within the right kidney in a patient with pyelonephritis.

Renal tract calculi

- Peak incidence 20–55 years, with a male: female preponderance of 4:1.
- Calculi form by crystallization of minerals in urine in the pelvicalyceal system. The most common are Ca^{2+} based. Associations include dehydration, UTI, metabolic abnormality, small bowel resection, and can be familial.

Clinical presentation

- Loin pain radiating to the groin, which can cause nausea.
- Haematuria (often microscopic) ± UTI.

Imaging

Plain film

90% of stone are visible (Ca^{2+}), (struvate (Mg^{2+} based) may not be). Plain films and IVU are becoming obsolete with the high sensitivity and availability of CT.

Ultrasound

Identifies hydronephrosis, indicative of obstruction. Calculi may be seen as the cause of obstruction. They are characteristic by the fact they cast an 'acoustic shadow'; however, small calculi may not do this, and maybe missed.

CT (Fig. 16.12)

Gaining popularity is the CT 'KUB' or CT 'stone chaser'. This is a non-IV contrast-enhanced CT scan covering the kidneys, ureters, and bladder. Performed prone with a full bladder. All stones with the exception of those produced by antiretroviral therapy are well seen. Upper tract obstruction may be seen. Alternative diagnosis may be found, such as appendicitis or diverticulitis.

IVU

Performed as a series of films. The acute protocol involves a control film and a film 10 minutes post-IV contrast, to identify obstruction.

Percutaneous nephrolithotomy (PCNL)

Performed in theatre by urologists with a radiologist. A retrograde ureterogram is performed to define the anatomy and the renal collecting system is punctured, like in a nephrostomy insertion, using ultrasound. The track is dilated and a device is inserted to perform stone removal.

Information for the radiologist

Clinical signs, i.e. side of pain, haematuria, presence of sepsis.

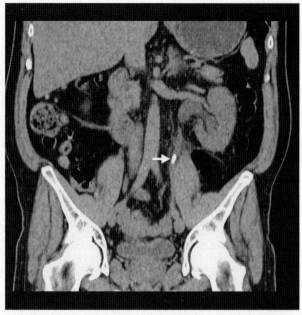

Fig. 16.12 Coronal CT showing left-sided hydronephrosis secondary to calculus within the upper left ureter (arrow).

Renal transplant dysfunction

Since the first successful renal transplant performed by Joseph Murray in 1954 between identical twins, transplant medicine has come a long way and with the advent of immunosuppressants, transplant surgery has become a hugely successful technique.

The majority of renal transplants are 'heterotopic' which means that they are transplanted to the patient with the native kidneys still *in situ*. Usually the patients will have had chronic renal failure for some time and their native kidneys will be small and sometimes difficult to see in detail. The transplant kidney is usually placed in one of the iliac fossae, outside the peritoneum.

Imaging

Ultrasound (Fig. 16.13)

Ultrasound is used to assess dilatation of the pelvicalyceal system (PCS), interlobar artery flow, to guide biopsy and interventions such as drainage of collections and placement of nephrostomy tubes. Ultrasound is also useful in assessment of postoperative complications including:

- Obstruction: a small degree of collecting system dilatation can be normal but persisting or worsening dilatation may indicate obstruction. This may be due to clot or debris within the ureter or as a result of an ischaemic-related stricture at the vesico-ureteric anastomosis. Nephrostomy under ultrasound guidance may be needed to relieve the obstruction in some circumstances.
- Vascular occlusion: ultrasound is used to assess the flow in the main renal artery and veins and in the interlobar arteries. This is done using Doppler ultrasound. An absent renal vein flow may indicate total occlusion whereas a partial occlusion will manifest as reverse end diastolic flow in the arterial Doppler trace.
- Rejection: non-specific ultrasound appearances include generalized oedema of the kidney and prominent pyramids. Clinical correlation is essential, and often biopsy is needed.

Information for the radiologist

Transplant anatomy, renal function, and signs of sepsis.

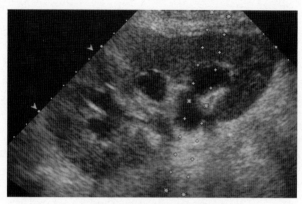

Fig. 16.13 Ultrasound showing hydronephrosis in a transplant kidney.

Vesico-ureteric reflux

- Predominantly affects children, with retrograde flow of urine from the bladder into ureters.
- Primary: majority of cases. Failure of the one-way vesico-ureteric valve.
- Secondary: to obstruction or poor functioning of the lower tract, e.g. posterior urethral valves or neurogenic bladder.
- May lead to renal scarring, hypertension, and chronic renal failure.
- See Table 16.3 for classification.

Table 16.3 International classification of radiographic grading of vesico-ureteric reflux

Grade I	Ureter only
Grade II	Ureter, pelvis, and calyces; no dilatation, normal calyceal fornices
Grade III	Mild or moderate dilatation and/or tortuosity of the ureter and mild or moderate dilatation of the renal pelvis. None/slight blunting of the fornices
Grade IV	Moderate dilatation and/or tortuosity of the ureter and moderate dilatation of the renal pelvis and calyces. Complete obliteration of the sharp angle of the fornices but maintenance of the papillary impressions in the majority of calyces
Grade V	Gross dilatation and tortuosity of the ureter. Gross dilatation of the renal pelvis and calyces. The papillary impressions are no longer visible in the majority of calyces

Clinical presentation

Usually diagnosed in investigation of antenatal hydronephrosis and paediatric UTI.

Imaging

Ultrasound

First-line investigation in UTI or suspected reflux, and for follow-up of antenatally diagnosed hydronephrosis. Local protocols vary, most units image children under 5 with a history of UTI, boys of any age with UTI, and children of any age with febrile UTI. Ultrasound features indicating vesico-ureteric reflux (VUR) include hydronephrosis, dilated distal ureters, small kidneys, renal scarring, and even demonstration of reflux in to the urinary tract during the examination. A normal ultrasound does not exclude VUR.

MCUG (Fig. 16.14)

Considered the gold standard investigation. Usually reserved for children under the age of 1 year due to the invasive nature of the procedure. Contrast is instilled into the bladder via a catheter and the ureters imaged during voiding for retrograde passage of contrast/dilatation. The urethra is also imaged in boys for signs of posterior urethral valves as a cause of VUR.

Nuclear medicine

Alternative technique to MCUG using 99m-pertechnetate instilled into the bladder. Advantage is reduced radiation dose but the limitations are lack of visualization of the urethral anatomy and difficulty in diagnosing minimal reflux as this may be obscured by bladder uptake. Technetium-99m dimer-captosuccinic acid (DMSA) is widely used in the investigation of VUR to diagnose and monitor renal scarring.

Information for the radiologist

- History of proven UTI.
- Previous imaging results including antenatal ultrasound scans.

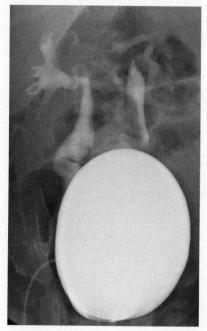

Fig. 16.14 Coronal image from micturating cystogram showing contrast from the bladder refluxing up both ureters into the kidneys.

Ectopic pregnancy

- Ectopic pregnancy occurs when the fertilized egg implants outside of the endometrium of the uterus.
- Incidence is 2% and the mortality rate is around 9–14%.
- Risk factors include previous ectopic pregnancy, pelvic inflammatory disease, tubal surgery and the use of intrauterine devices.

Clinical presentation

Abdominal pain and vaginal spotting following a period of amenorrhea. Indirect signs of ruptured ectopic are hypovolaemic shock, and shoulder tip pain due to diaphragmatic irritation. Pain may decrease after rupture.

Imaging

Imaging should only be performed in stable patients. Initial evaluation of ectopic pregnancy should include a TV ultrasound (Fig. 16.15) in conjunction with a serum βhCG level. If the features of a normal pregnancy are not identified at a certain βhCG level, then close scrutiny for an ectopic pregnancy required (Table 16.4).

Table 16.4 Correlation of βhCG, gestational age, and TVUS findings

	βhCG level (mIU/ml)	Gestational age (weeks)
Gestational sac	2000	4.5
Yolk sac	7000	5
Fetal pole	11000	5–6
Fetal heart beat	25000	5–6

Ultrasound

95% of ectopic pregnancies are tubal. Findings include:
- An adnexal mass: size of mass, the presence of a gestational sac, a fetal pole, heart beat, and a yolk sac.
- Pregnancy in a non-specific adnexal mass.
- Pelvic fluid: look in the pouch of Douglas and right posterior subhepatic space.
- The endometrium which may be normal or there may be a pseudogestation sac.

MRI

Problem solving modality to confirm or better define suspected ectopic pregnancy. Looking for:
- An extrauterine gestational sac.
- Fresh haematoma.
- Tubal wall enhancement post contrast, due to increased vascularity following implantation.

Information for the radiologist
- Salient history and examination findings.
- Last menstrual period important.
- βhCG level if known.

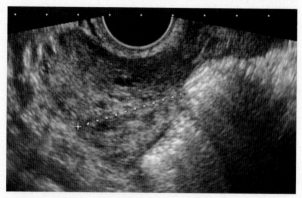

Fig. 16.15 Image from a TV ultrasound showing a complex mass (indicated by callipers) inseparable from the right ovary. This was confirmed at surgery to be a tubal ectopic pregnancy, and the patient underwent a salpingo-oophorectomy.

Endometriosis

This is the presence of endometrial glands and stroma outside the uterine cavity and musculature. Ectopic endometrial material responds to hormonal stimuli causing cyclical haemorrhage. Common sites for endometrial deposits include the ovaries and pelvic peritoneum. Deep endometriosis describes endometriosis that infiltrates the peritoneum >5mm. These deposits are found in the subperitoneal pelvic space, the uterosacral ligaments, rectovaginal septum, and also in the bladder and bowel wall.

Clinical presentation

Many patients are asymptomatic. It commonly presents with infertility or pelvic pain.

Imaging

Ultrasound and MRI are the most useful tests. Occasionally the diagnosis may be unsuspected, and suggests following other imaging, such as barium enema showing endometrial serosal deposits on the bowel wall, typically at the rectosigmoid.

Ultrasound

- Endometriomas ('chocolate cysts') appear as complex cystic ovarian mass with homogeneous low level echoes and a thick wall (Fig. 16.16).
- Hydrosalpinx maybe present.
- Assessment of superficial peritoneal deposits, ovarian foci and deep endometriosis is less accurate with ultrasound.

MRI

- Typical MRI features of endometriomas include high signal intensity on T1-weighted sequences due to blood products in the cyst. There may be layering of fluid within the cyst due to blood products of different ages.
- Features of deep endometriosis depend on whether it is infiltrative small implants, visceral implants, or solid deep lesions in the posterior cul-de-sac. Secondary complications of adhesions, such as bowel obstruction may be seen.

Information for the radiologist

Detailed clinical symptoms and examination findings will help the radiologist identify endometriotic deposits accurately particularly when the deposits are small and subtle.

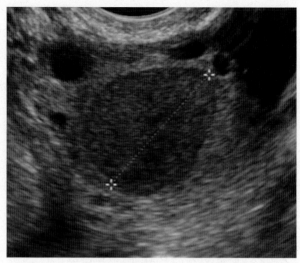

Fig. 16.16 Ultrasound showing endometrioma within the right ovary.

Ovarian torsion

- The abnormal rotation of the ovary on its vascular pedicle, compromising the venous and arterial blood supply to the ovary.
- Predisposing factors include: ovarian cyst (>5cm) or cystic neoplasm, cystic ovaries associated with ovarian hyperstimulation syndrome and polycystic ovaries.
- Initially the venous outflow and lymphatic drainage are compromised, with maintenance of arterial inflow. The ovary enlarges and becomes oedematous causing arterial thrombosis, leading to ovarian ischaemia and infarction.
- Highest prevalence is in women of reproductive age. 17–20% of cases occur in pregnant women.

Clinical presentation

Symptoms may be non-specific—lower abdominal pain, nausea and vomiting associated with tenderness/peritonism, ± a palpable mass. Pain may be intermittent.

Imaging

Ultrasound

First-line investigation. Both TA and TV ultrasound should be performed.
- A unilateral enlarged ovary ± a coexistent ovarian mass.
- Peripheral ovarian follicles ('string of pearl' sign) as the follicles are displaced by the oedematous stroma.
- Free fluid in pelvis.
- Arterial and venous blood flow can be maintained despite a twisted vascular pedicle; however, absence of blood flow is highly suggestive of the diagnosis.

CT (Fig. 16.17a)

May be performed prior to ultrasound, as CT is commonly used as the first-line investigation for non-specific abdominal and pelvic pain.
- An adnexal mass which may be displaced to the midline.
- Ascites or haemoperitoneum.
- Reduced central enhancement of the ovary.
- Haemorrhage and gas in the ovary if necrotic.
- Stranding and inflammatory changes in the adjacent fat.

MRI (Fig. 16.17b)

May be required when pelvic ultrasound inconclusive.

Information for the radiologist

- Last menstrual period—is the patient pregnant?
- Is there any relevant gynaecological history?
- Is the woman taking infertility drugs?
- Are there any other symptoms to suggest other diagnoses, e.g. diverticulitis, appendicitis?

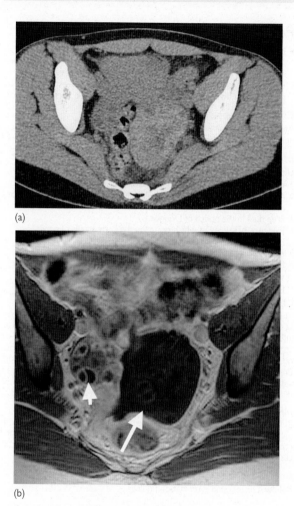

(a)

(b)

Fig. 16.17 a) CT and b) MRI in a patient with left-sided ovarian torsion. The CT shows a bulky, high attenuation left ovary, in keeping with haemorrhage. MRI showing enlarged, low signal intensity infarcted left ovary (long arrow), showing no enhancement compared to the normal right ovary (short arrow).

Pelvic inflammatory disease

- Infection of the upper genital tract, commonly sexually transmitted *Chlamydia trachomatis* or *Neisseria gonorrhoeae*. Less commonly occurs as a result of secondary infection from appendicitis or diverticulitis.
- Peak incidence rate is in women aged 20–24 years. Long-term sequelae include infertility, ectopic pregnancy, and chronic pain if left untreated.

Clinical presentation

Abdominal pain, raised temperature, vaginal discharge, abdominal tenderness, cervical and adnexal tenderness.

Imaging

Ultrasound (Fig. 16.18)

TA and TV ultrasound are the first-line investigations, looking for:

- An enlarged and indistinct uterus. Adjacent fat may be inflamed and of increased echogenicity.
- Free fluid in the pouch of Douglas.
- Evidence of salpingitis which occurs in the early stages of pelvic inflammatory disease (PID).
- A tubo-ovarian complex/abscess.
- Perihepatitis: Fitz–Hugh–Curtis syndrome occurs when inflammatory exudates spread to the liver via the right paracolic gutter from the pelvis, causing RUQ pain.

CT

This may be the first investigation if symptoms are non-specific. Advantages of CT over US are that firstly, it is easier to appreciate the effects of pelvic inflammation on adjacent structures, e.g. bowel ileus, hydroureter, or appendicitis. Secondly, subtle signs of inflammation are easier to appreciate on CT, e.g. there may be haziness in the pre-sacral fat, thickening of the uterosacral ligaments, peritoneal enhancement or periovarian stranding in adjacent fat. Classic features of PID are also appreciated on CT such as dilated fallopian tubes, adnexal abscesses, enlarged ovaries, and free fluid.

MRI

MRI has a higher sensitivity and specificity in depicting PID compared with TV ultrasound. However, ultrasound is a relatively low cost and more readily accessible compared to MRI. MRI should only be used in difficult cases as a problem solver.

Information for the radiologist

Relevant history and examination findings.

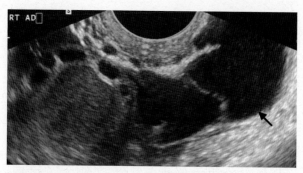

Fig. 16.18 Ultrasound showing dilated, fluid filled fallopian tube (arrow). The fluid is seen to contain debris.

Epididymitis

May be acute or chronic. Usually acute, secondary to infection, resolving with antibiotic therapy. The role of imaging is to confirm the diagnosis and exclude complications.

Clinical presentation

- *Acute epididymitis:* presentation is with acute pain and scrotal inflammation. Secondary to ascending UTI, sexually transmitted infection, or haematogenous infection. Recent instrumentation can be a factor. Numerous bacteria are associated, e.g. *Escherichia coli*, *Pseudomonas*, gonorrhoea, *Chlamydia*, and TB.
- *Chronic epididymitis:* pain and tenderness for >6 weeks, often unclear aetiology. Associations: previous infection, scrotal surgery, or systemic inflammatory conditions. Investigate for infection especially *Chlamydia*. Treatment is with antibiotics and anti-inflammatories. Role of imaging is limited.

Investigations

FBC (increased WCC) and urine sample. *Chlamydia* can be difficult to culture and may require prostatic massage or direct epididymal sampling.

Differential diagnosis

- Orchitis: if present without epididymitis is likely mumps.
- Sperm granuloma (post vasectomy).
- Torsion (younger age group).
- Tumour: especially in young children an extra-testicular mass in the scrotum may represent a rhabdomyosarcoma.

Imaging

Ultrasound (Fig. 16.19)

Performed with a high-frequency probe. In acute epididymitis the entire epididymis is enlarged, occasionally only the head. The echogenicity is either low due to oedema or heterogeneous. Blood flow is mostly increased. Complications include scrotal abscesses. The collection should demonstrate increased through transmission of sound (picture looks brighter behind)—an important ultrasound imaging sign. Alternative pathology can be demonstrated such as tumour or orchitis.

In chronic epididymitis the imaging can be normal or a more subtle swelling of the epididymis may be seen.

Information for the radiologist

Clinical history, in particular any surgical procedures.

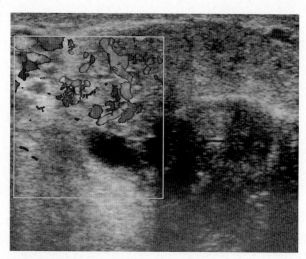

Fig. 16.19 Ultrasound showing oedematous hyperaemic epididymitis in a patient with epididymitis.

Testicular torsion

- Male <30 years, peak 10–14 years.
- Associated with bell clapper insertion of the testis within the tunica vaginalis, allowing the spermatic cord to wind around with resultant vascular compromise.

Clinical presentation

Presentation is with pain severe enough to inhibit mobility and cause nausea. The testis can occasionally un-tort and re-tort, giving an episodic history of pain. The differential diagnosis is of a torted hydatid of Morgagni (testicular appendage) and infection (epididymitis/orchitis). History and examination help differentiate. Typically the torted testis will be exquisitely tender and have a high horizontal lie in an inflamed scrotum. Boys at the younger end of the spectrum can present with abdominal pain and nausea.

⚠ Acute torsion of the testis is a surgical emergency which requires urgent operative exploration with bilateral orchidopexy (if viable) or orchidectomy and contralateral orchidopexy (if non-viable). Do not waste time requesting an ultrasound or nuclear scan to assess for viability. Early restoration of blood supply is the aim.

Imaging

Ultrasound (Fig. 16.20)

Performed when other causes of scrotal pain are suspected such as epidimyo-orchitis or when the history of torsion is of such chronicity that the test is to confirm the presence of a non-viable testis.

If scanned in acute torsion the affected testis will be swollen, of low echogenicity, and a reactive hydrocoele may be present. There may be no Doppler blood flow seen, or reactive hyperaemia. The presence of peripheral flow around the testis is a poor prognostic indicator and increases over time. In the non-viable testis no central blood flow will be detected and peripheral flow is usually identified. The echogenicity will be heterogeneous. False negative and false positive results are not uncommon. Clinical acumen is of the highest importance.

Nuclear perfusion scan

Technetium-99m pertechnitate IV injection has a role in determining the presence of non-viable testis in cases with a suggestive chronicity of symptoms, but not in the acute setting.

Information for the radiologist

Clinical history, especially length of symptoms.

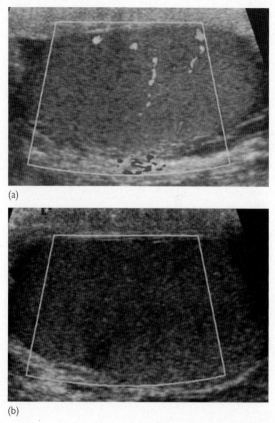

(a)

(b)

Fig. 16.20 Two ultrasound images from a patient with unilateral testicular torsion. The first image a) is from the normal testis, showing normal echogenicity (brightness) and colour flow. The second image b) is from the symptomatic side, showing the torted testicle that is swollen, hypoechoic (darker), with no colour flow compared to the normal side.

Musculoskeletal differential diagnosis

Moth-eaten bone

- Neoplastic:
  - Metastases.
  - Multiple myeloma.
  - Leukaemia.
  - Primary bone tumours, e.g. sarcoma.
  - Langerhans cell histiocytosis.
- Infection:
  - Acute osteomyelitis.

Osteopenia

- Osteoporosis.
- Osteomalacia.
- Hyperparathyroidism.
- Diffuse infiltrative bone disease.

Increased uptake on bone scans

- Metastases.
- Joint disease.
- Traumatic fractures.
- Post surgery: up to 1 year.
- Infection.
- Paget's disease.
- Superscan.
- Metabolic bone disease.

Scoliosis

- Idiopathic.
- Congenital.
- Neuropathic.
- Neuromuscular disorders.
- Neuroectodermal diseases.
- Post radiotherapy.
- Leg-length discrepancy.

Musculoskeletal presenting syndromes

Bone pain

This may be local or general. Pain may also be referred, and a non-specific symptom. Certain features may be more worrying, e.g. pain causing the patient to wake up from sleep.

Causes
- Skeletal:
  - Fracture/trauma.
  - Primary bone tumour (benign or malignant).
  - Infection.
  - Metastases.
  - Joint disease.
- Soft tissue:
  - Infection.
  - Trauma.
  - Tumour.
  - Foreign body.

Imaging

This depends on the history and location of symptoms. For bony pathology, plain radiographs are the first-line imaging modality. For investigation of soft tissue pathology, ultrasound is better, and if non-conclusive, MRI as second line.

Plain film

Good for detection of fractures, bony lesions, and established osteomyelitis. (Radiographs may be normal in early osteomyelitis.)

Ultrasound

For identification of collections within the soft tissues, identification of certain foreign bodies, and traumatic soft tissue injuries.

MRI

Most sensitive investigation, but expensive and limited availability. Good for bony pathology and soft tissues tumours, injury, and infection.

Nuclear medicine

Bone scan can be useful if pain is persistent and initial investigations unhelpful, or if multifocal pathology.

Swollen joint

In the acute presentation, it is important to exclude septic arthritis, as this can lead to joint destruction if left untreated.

Causes
- Trauma:
  - Effusion/haemarthrosis.
- Infection:
  - Septic arthritis.
  - Osteomyelitis.
- Inflammation:
  - Synovitis.
  - Bursitis.
  - Rheumatoid arthritis.
  - Gout.
  - Osteoarthritis.
- Tumour:
  - Primary bone tumours.
  - Metastases.
- Haematological conditions:
  - Sickle call anaemia.
  - Haemophilia.

Imaging

Plain film
Plain films are usually the first-line investigation. They may be normal in infection, and joint aspiration may be needed to exclude or prove joint infection.

Ultrasound
This is used to identify effusions, to guide aspiration in certain cases, and can show synovial hypertrophy.

MRI
Good for identification of effusions, ligament and tendon disruption, fractures. Also sensitive in assessment of bony tumour extension, synovial hypertrophy, and marrow abnormalities.

Soft tissue lump

Common benign causes

- Lipoma.
- Lymphadenopathy (commonly normal prominent nodes).
- Haematoma.
- Haemangioma/AVM.
- Neurofibroma.
- Abscess.
- Ganglion cyst (close to joint).

Common malignant causes

- Metastatic soft tissue deposits.
- Lymphadenopathy (lymphoma/malignant involvement).
- Sarcomatous lesions.

Imaging

Plain film

May detect associated bony destruction, or calcification within the soft tissues.

Ultrasound

Most valuable imaging modality in soft tissue pathology. Allows identification and characterization of mass and, if indicated, image-guided biopsy. Deeper lesions may be difficult to see.

MRI

The most sensitive modality. Good for characterization, and can look at enhancement using gadolinium.

Bony lesions

The patient's age, symptoms, and past medical history are the primary clues in the assessment of bone tumours.

Benign bone tumour

- Bone cyst.
- Non-ossifying fibroma.
- Giant cell tumour.
- Infection.

Malignant bone tumour

- Metastases.
- Multiple myeloma/plasmocytoma.
- Sarcoma (Ewing's, osteosarcoma, chondrosarcoma).
- Lymphoma/leukaemia.

Imaging

The role of imaging is to decide if the lesion has benign or aggressive features. If malignant in appearance, imaging can show the local extent, assess for distant metastases, and aid biopsy, if indicated. Biopsy of primary bone tumours is performed only after discussion with radiologists, and may involve the patient being refereed to a tertiary bone referral centre.

Plain film

- Identify bony lesions, associated fractures and marrow involvement.

Ultrasound

- Limited use in bony pathology.

CT

- Used sometimes in characterization of lesions, and if malignant for detection of distant metastases.

MRI

- Show local extent of tumour, and characteristics.

Nuclear medicine

- Bone scan used to detect other foci of bony involvement.

Musculoskeletal conditions

Osteoarthritis

A chronic disease characterized by cartilage degeneration in synovial joints. Affects 80–90% of people over the age of 65 years.[1] Usually caused by 'wear and tear' but may also result from:

- Normal forces on abnormal joints, e.g. slipped upper femoral epiphyses.
- Abnormal forces on normal joints, e.g. obesity causing osteoarthritis (OA) of the knees.

Clinical presentation

Patients present with joint pain. On examination, they have stiff joints with reduced range of movement and bony deformity around the joints. Unlike rheumatoid arthritis, there is often asymmetry between sides.

Imaging

Plain film

This is the preferred imaging modality. The cardinal features are:

- Loss of joint space.
- Subchondral sclerosis.
- Subchondral cysts.
- Osteophytes (bone spurs) (Fig. 19.1).

The disease distribution can be useful to distinguish OA from other the arthritides:

- Hands: distal interphalangeal joints (DIPJs) >proximal interphalangeal joint (PIPJs), thumb carpometacarpal joints (CMCJs), metacarpophalangeal joints (MCPJs), and the trapezio-scaphoid joint.
- Feet: similar to hand.
- Hip: superior joint space narrowing at the maximum weight-bearing joint area.
- Knee: medial compartment most commonly affected due to weight distribution.
- Spine: apophyseal joints, narrowing of intervertebral disc spaces.
- Sacroiliac joints (SIJs): contralateral SIJ to the arthritic hip joint.

MRI

This can be used as a specialist investigation to look for early loss of joint cartilage, usually in the hips or knees.

Information for the radiologist

- Site, duration, and severity of patient's symptoms.
- Predisposing factors to OA, e.g. obesity, acromegaly, avascular necrosis, slipped upper femoral epiphyses, previous trauma, or joint infections.

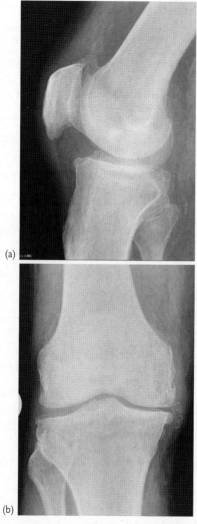

Fig. 19.1 Images a) and b) show severe OA of the knee with marginal osteophytes, loss of joint cartilage, and subchondral sclerosis.

Reference

1 Roberts J, Burch TA. Osteoarthritis prevalence in adults by age, sex, race, and geographic area. *Vital Health Stat 1.* 1966; **11**(15):1–27.

Rheumatoid arthritis

This is a chronic systemic disorder causing a bilateral symmetrical inflammatory joint disease. Affects women >men, usually aged between 40–60 at diagnosis. Synovial joints are affected with synovial hyperaemia and proliferation (pannus) leading to bone erosions and cartilage destruction.

Clinical presentation

The American Rheumatism Association decree that at least 4 of the following criteria are required, lasting at least 6 weeks, for diagnosis:[1]

- Early morning joint stiffness, which lasts 1 hour before improvement.
- Simultaneous joint swelling in at least 3 joints.
- Symmetrical arthritis involving in particular the PIPJs, MCPJs, or wrist.
- Subcutaneous nodules.
- Positive rheumatoid factor (above 95th percentile).
- Typical radiographic changes of erosions and periarticular osteopenia.

Imaging

Plain film

Appearances may be normal. Early signs include periarticular osteopenia, subcortical synovial cysts, soft tissue swelling, and widened joint spaces due to synovial inflammation. Later signs include erosions, reduction in joint space secondary to cartilage destruction, joint subluxation, ankylosis and loose bodies.

- Hand (Fig. 19.2a): affects MCPJs and PIPJs >DIPJs. Characteristic deformities include:
  - Ulnar deviation at the wrist.
  - Ankylosis of the carpal bones.
  - Boutonniere: hyperflexion at PIPJ, hyperextension at DIPJ.
  - Swan-neck: hyperextension at PIPJ, hyperflexion at DIPJ.
  - Mallet finger: droopy distal phalanx.
- Feet: similar appearances to the hands.
- Cervical spine: erosions of the odontoid peg and atlanto-axial subluxation.
- Shoulder: involves the glenohumeral and acromioclavicular joints (Fig. 19.2b).
- Knees: bilateral and symmetrical. Osteoporosis and erosions.
- Chest: pleural or pericardial effusions, rheumatoid nodules which may cavitate and occasionally lower zone fibrosis.

Ultrasound

May demonstrate synovitis, joint effusions and tendon rupture.

MRI

Demonstrates synovitis, erosive changes, and pannus.

Information for the radiologist

- Distribution and duration of symptoms.
- Rheumatoid factor if known.

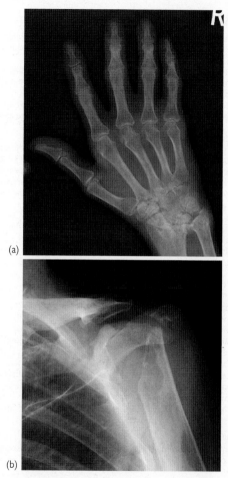

Fig. 19.2 A 55-year-old patient with severe right hand and left shoulder deformity. a) Demonstrates severe erosive disease primarily affecting the radio-carpal, carpal and metacarpalphalangeal joints. b) Shows complete loss of the humeral head as well as severe erosive disease to the acromio-clavicular joint.

Reference

1 Arnett F, Edworthy S, Bloch DA, *et al.* The American Rheumatism Association 1987 revised criteria for the classification of rheumatoid arthritis. *Arthritis Rheum* 1987; **31**(3):315–24.

Crystal deposition

- Gout: deposition of monosodium urate crystals in and around joints or in the urinary tract. Predominantly affects middle aged/elderly men. Serum uric acid is often raised.
- Calcium pyrophosphate deposition disease (CPPD): deposition of calcium pyrophosphate crystals in and around joints. Commonly associated with gout.
- Alkaptonuria: rare autosomal recessive disorder causing excess homogentisic acid deposition in connective tissues, cartilage and bone.

Clinical presentation

- Gout: usually monoarticular and may be asymptomatic in the early stages. Acute presentations are with a hot, swollen, painful joint, typically the first MCPJ. Chronic presentations are with repeated bouts of arthritis in the same joint. Less common presentations are with urinary calculi (radiolucent), tendon rupture or paraesthesia due to nerve paralysis.
- CPPD: presentation may be similar to gout (pseudogout), OA or rheumatoid arthritis. Can be monoarticular or polyarticular and most commonly affects the knees, wrist, MCPJs, and PIPJs.
- Alkaptonuria: back pain, skin and sclera pigmentation, dark urine, heart failure, or renal failure.

Imaging

Plain film

In the early stages often normal.

- Gout: affects feet >hands and small joints >large joints. Soft tissue swelling, 'punched-out' erosions with overhanging edges, subchondral cysts and soft tissue crystal deposition which may calcify (gouty tophi) (Fig. 19.3).
- CPPD: resembles OA with osteophyte formation, joint space narrowing, subchondral cysts, and sclerosis. Cartilage calcification (chondrocalcinosis) is characteristic, especially around the knee, pubic symphysis, and triangular fibrocartilage of the wrist.
- Alkaptonuria: calcification of intervertebral discs, vertebral ankylosis and osteophytosis. Early onset OA is also a feature.

Ultrasound

May identify soft tissue calcification, synovitis, nerve compression, tendon rupture or renal calculi.

CT

Used to identify radiolucent urinary calculi.

MRI

Not commonly used. Will show erosions, soft tissue calcification, synovitis and bony ankylosis.

Information for the radiologist

- Site, duration and frequency of symptoms.
- Serum urate if known.

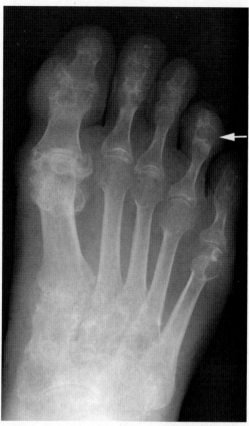

Fig. 19.3 Single foot radiograph taken after a 45-year-old presented with an exquisitely painful, red great toe with no history of preceding trauma. There is widespread degenerative change with multiple punched out para-articular erosions (arrow) and marked soft tissue swelling. These findings are typical for gout.

Ankylosing spondylitis

This is an autoimmune seronegative disease, affecting ligamentous insertions, synovial and cartilaginous joints. It causes a chronic arthritis eventually leading to bony ankylosis and enthesopathy, classically involving the spine, pelvis, proximal femur, and calcaneus.

Clinical presentation

The typical patient is a young Caucasian adult male (15–35 years). They present with insidious onset of lower back pain and stiffness, usually worse in the mornings. As ankylosis progresses, the range of movement reduces. Complications include fractures, pulmonary fibrosis, and respiratory compromise. Other associations include aortic valve incompetence, iritis, and ulcerative colitis.

Imaging

Plain film (Fig. 19.4a)

These are good for monitoring progression.

- SIJs: indistinct joint margins are followed by sclerosis and later ankylosis. Usually bilateral and symmetrical.
- Spine: changes usually begin in the lumbar spine:
  - 'Bamboo spine' (flowing syndesmophytes on the AP radiograph).
  - Ossification of spinous ligaments.
  - Squaring of anterior vertebral end-plates (Romanus lesions).
  - 'Shiny corner' of vertebral bodies secondary to sclerosis.
  - Apophyseal erosions and ankylosis.
  - Disc calcification.
  - Kyphosis.
  - Atlanto-axial subluxation.
- Hands: osteophytes, osteoporosis, joint space narrowing and erosions affecting the MCPJ, PIPJ, DIPJ's.
- Chest: upper lobe fibrosis, occasional bullae and cavitation.
- Other: periostitic 'whiskering' at sites of ligamentous insertions, e.g. greater femoral trochanter, iliac crest, ischial tuberosity, calcaneum.

CT

HRCT chest may show upper lobe fibrosis, peripheral interstitial lung disease, and bronchiectasis.

MRI (Fig. 19.4b)

This has an expanding role in the early detection of ankylosing spondylitis. The earliest findings are of low-grade oedema to the SIJs and the corners of the vertebral bodies (the entheses).

Information for the radiologist

- Presenting symptoms including sites of pain/tenderness.
- HLA-B27 status if available (95% of patients are carriers).
- Any history or clinical signs indicating UC, aortic valve disease, iritis, or pulmonary fibrosis.

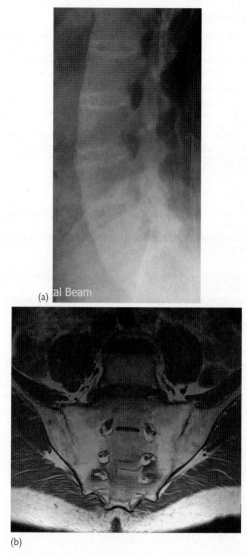

(a) al Beam

(b)

Fig. 19.4 A 40-year-old male with stiffness in the back. a) Lateral lumbar spine radiograph showing smooth fusion of all the lumbar vertebral bodies. b) T1-weighted sacral MRI showing complete ankylosis of the SIJs consistent with ankylosing spondylitis.

Degenerative disc disease

Degenerative disc disease is mechanical degeneration of the intervertebral discs of the spine. This can lead to a prolapsed or herniated disc. About 90% of all disc prolapses occur at the L4/L5 and L5/S1 levels although the cervical spine can also be affected.

Clinical presentation

- Non-specific back pain.
- May present with radiation to the side of the disc prolapse if there is nerve root compression.
- Motor symptoms develop as the disc compresses the nerve further.
- Cauda equine syndrome is a combination of saddle (perineal anaesthesia), para-paresis, loss of bowel and bladder control due to a central disc prolapse compressing the cauda equine.

Imaging

Plain film

- Plain radiographs are often the first modality used, although they are of limited value.
- They may show a reduction in disc height and degenerative changes affecting the facet joints.

CT

- CT is only used where MRI is contraindicated such as patients with aneurysm clips or severe claustrophobics.
- CT may show a disc prolapse on careful review but it is of more value showing degenerative facet joints.
- Definitive diagnosis can be made by instilling contrast into the CSF—known as a CT myelogram. This defines the prolapsed disc.

MRI

- MRI is the modality of choice for imaging of suspected disc prolapse.
- The prolapsed disc can be visualized and any compression of the nerve can be seen.
- Standard sets of images include sagittal and axial T1 and T2 sequences.
- The nomenclature for disc prolapse has been standardized (Table 19.1).

Information for the radiologist

- The dermatome, myotomes, and side of affected areas.
- Any associated neurology.
- Any signs of cauda equine syndrome.
- History of previous trauma, surgery to the spine or malignancy.

Table 19.1 Nomenclature defined by North American Spine Society in 2001

Name	Meaning
Disc herniation	Localized displacement of disc material beyond the intervertebral disc space
Bulge	Disc between 50–100% circumferentially beyond the edges—not a form of herniation
Broad-based disc	Disc displaced between 25–50% circumferentially beyond the edges
Focal	Disc displaced <25% of the circumference
Protrusion	Disc material is focally displaced
Extrusion	Displaced disc material has a greater length than width
Sequestration	Disc material has lost continuity with the parent disc

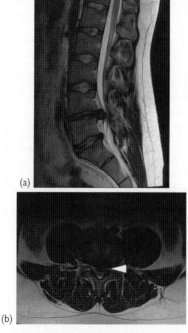

(a)

(b)

Fig. 19.5 A 35-year-old patient with sudden onset severe left sided sciatica.
a) Sagittal T2-weighted image showing extrusion of the L4/5 intervertebral disc.
b) Axial T2-weighted image showing the full extent of this (arrowhead).

Cord compression

This is a surgical emergency secondary to compression of the spinal cord by tumour, pus, blood, bone, or disc material. This requires decompression to prevent a long-term neurological deficit.

Clinical presentation

Patients complain of back pain, paralysis below the level of compression, urinary and faecal incontinence.

Imaging

Timing of imaging

Urgent imaging is indicated as once complete paralysis has been present for >24 hours then the chance of any reasonable recovery decreases dramatically. However, there is no reason to scan someone in the middle of the night unless a surgeon is available who can operate immediately. It is much more appropriate to get the scan done first thing in the morning in time for the day-time emergency lists.

Plain film

These are helpful in showing areas of vertebral collapse or fracture but they cannot show what is causing the cord compression.

MRI (Fig. 19.6)

Other imaging modalities may provide useful information about trauma and vertebral collapse but MRI is the investigation of choice. This demonstrates what is causing the compression and over how much of a distance. Cord signal change is helpful and in trauma the presence of blood within the cord is a bad prognostic sign. In addition this will provide detail about other abnormalities in the region and give the surgeon a road-map for any planned surgery.

CT myelography

In patients who have contraindications for MRI then this is an alternative. Iodine dye is introduced into the dural sac using fluoroscopic control. CT is then used to look for indirect evidence of obstruction i.e. is there a level where the dye cannot pass through.

Information for the radiologist

- Does the patient have any known malignancy?
- Has the patient had any recent surgery—the risk of spinal infection is much higher where there has been recent thoracic or abdominal surgery?
- Is the patient on any form of anticoagulation?

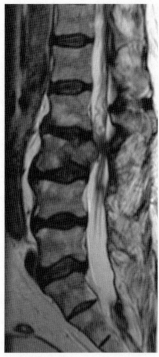

Fig. 19.6 A 66-year-old male with sudden urinary incontinence. This shows collapse of the L3 vertebral body secondary to tumour replacement of the body. This is impinging upon the cauda equina and leading to severe nerve compression.

Osteomyelitis

Osteomyelitis is a debilitating condition with a considerable morbidity. It affects both children and adults, albeit differently.

In children, the commonest route is by haematogenous spread. Infection typically localizes to the metaphysis with the lower limbs usually affected. The most common organism is *Staphylococcus aureus*. Chronic infection can lead to a Brodie's abscess.

In adults the commonest causes are direct inoculation or pre-existing conditions such as diabetes. *Staphylococcus aureus* and streptococci are the most commonly isolated organisms. Joint involvement is common. Chronic osteomyelitis in adulthood is usually due to a foreign body, chronic underlying disease, or previous trauma.

Clinical presentation

- Fever, malaise, lethargy, and weight loss.
- In children, there may be a history of recent infection.
- In adults, there may be a previous history of surgery or IV drug abuse.

Imaging

Plain film

- Plain films can be insensitive in the early phase (there has to be 50% loss of bone before there is an appreciable radiographic change).
- Ill defined lucency at the site of infection. In children this is usually at the metaphysis of the bone.
- Periosteal elevation is seen later.
- Chronic osteomyelitis is often characterized by necrotic bone termed a 'sequestrum'.

Bone scintigraphy

- Osteomyelitis causes increased osteoblastic activity, which shows up as an area of increased uptake.
- Scintigraphy can therefore be used to confirm areas of active infection and identify if there are multiple foci.

CT

CT is useful in identifying periosteal elevation, sequestra, or foreign bodies.

MRI (Fig. 19.7)

- MRI is the modality of choice for further investigation of osteomyelitis.
- It can identify early oedema, periosteal reaction, soft tissue collections, and sequestra at the site of infection.

Information for the radiologist

- Area of concern.
- Past history of immunosuppression, chronic disease, IV drug abuse, surgery, and trauma.
- Inflammatory markers.

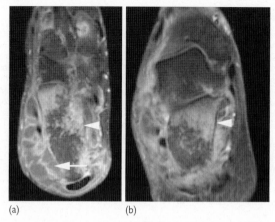

(a)   (b)

Fig. 19.7 A 20-year-old patient admitted with red and grossly swollen hindfoot. Figures 19.7a and 19.7b are T1-weighted gadolinium axial images of the hindfoot showing osteomyelitis of the calcaneus (arrowheads) and soft tissue pus (arrow).

Discitis

Discitis is infection of the intervertebral discs. It accounts for 2–4% of all skeletal infection with a male:female ratio of 3:1. There are 2 distinct affected age groups: children and adults aged >50. The infection may be confined to a single disc space or multiple levels with the lumbar spine commonly affected. The most commonly isolated pathogen is *Staphylococcus aureus* (60%) although other organisms including TB should always be considered. The three main routes of infection are: haematogenous (commonest), direct inoculation (iatrogenic), or contiguous spread. Discitis may progress to give vertebral body osteomyelitis.

Clinical presentation

- Red flag signs (see Box 19.1) for spinal pathology.
- Acute, non-traumatic localized pain.
- Non-specific symptoms including fever, weight loss, and malaise.
- Chronic illnesses such as diabetes and immunosuppression predispose to it.

Box 19.1 Red flag signs for spinal pathology

- Age of onset <20 or >50 years
- Thoracic pain
- Fever and unexplained with loss
- Bladder and bowel dysfunction
- History of carcinoma
- Ill health or previous medical illness
- Progressive neurological deficit
- Disturbed gait or saddle anaesthesia.

Imaging

Plain film
- This is relatively insensitive for early infection.
- Loss of disc space.
- Indistinct end plates.
- Chronic changes include end-plate sclerosis or collapse.
- Gradual disc obliteration and vertebral fusion.

CT
- CT is not routinely used in the initial work-up.
- It has a role in assessment of the bony anatomy, to guide biopsies, and where the patient cannot tolerate an MRI.

MRI
- MRI is the initial modality of choice.
- Standard sequences include T1-weighted, STIR and T1-weighted post-contrast sagittal and axial planes (Fig. 19.8).
- T1 images will show low signal intensity changes to the disc and vertebral body with loss of disc height.
- STIR images show high signal in the disc, adjacent vertebral end plates, and paravertebral soft tissues.

- Post-contrast T1 images show ring enhancement of pus and can be used to differentiate pus from oedema.

Information for the radiologist
- Predisposing factors such as recent surgery?
- What are the inflammatory markers?
- Is there any evidence of sepsis?

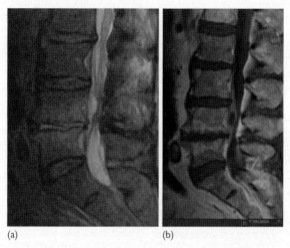

(a)   (b)

Fig. 19.8 A 56-year-old patient with severe low back pain 1 month after an aortic aneurysm repair. a) Sagittal STIR image demonstrating oedema to the L4/L5 intervertebral disc, oedema to both the L4 and L5 vertebral bodies and an epidural abscess at this level. b) T1 gadolinium image showing peripheral enhancement of the abscess.

Psoas abscess

The psoas is a retroperitoneal muscle that originates from the lateral borders of T12 to L5. It lies in close proximity to the sigmoid colon, appendix, ureters, iliac lymph nodes, and the spine. Psoas abscesses are a result of its rich vascular supply and by conditions affecting the adjacent structures (Table 19.2). Primary psoas abscesses are commonly seen in children whilst secondary are seen in adults, commonly in IV drug abusers.

Clinical presentation
- Non-specific abdominal pain/back pain.
- Pyrexia, malaise, and weight loss.
- Referred pain to the hips and femoral flexion.

Imaging
Plain film
This will not demonstrate a psoas abscess but it may point to the cause.

Ultrasound
Ultrasound can be used to identify a psoas abscess although it may not be able to demonstrate the underlying cause.

CT
- Post contrast-enhanced CT is the modality of choice as it can identify both a psoas abscess (a ring enhancing area) and its underlying cause.
- Both CT and ultrasound can be used to drain psoas abscesses percutaneously.

MRI (Fig. 19.9)
- MRI's good soft tissue resolution will demonstrate these well.
- MRI is superior to CT where there is an underlying spinal cause as it will clearly show spinal and epidural extension.

Information for the radiologist
- Clinical presentation.
- Inflammatory markers.
- Any previous chronic diseases such as diverticulosis or history of IV drug abuse.

Table 19.2 Predisposing causes for psoas abscess

Disease site	Conditions
GI tract	Diverticulitis, appendicitis, Crohns, colorectal cancer, appendiceal tumour
GU tract	UTI, extracorporeal shock wave lithotripsy, GU cancers
Musculoskeletal infections	Vertebral osteomyelitis, discitis, infectious sacro-ilitis, septic arthritis
Others	Endocarditis, femoral artery catheterization, endocarditis, infected abdominal aortic aneurysm, spinal surgery

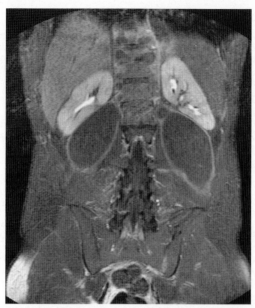

Fig. 19.9 Coronal T1 gadolinium image of the retroperitoneum demonstrating bilateral psoas abscesses.

Septic arthritis

This is one of the true orthopaedic emergencies where the joint requires washout on the same day. The reason for this is that active intra-articular infection very quickly results in cartilage lysis. This will then lead to premature OA and even ankylosis later on. This means that any imaging should be performed in a timely manner.

Clinical presentation

Patients with septic arthritis usually present with a swollen painful joint that they refuse to move. They will have raised inflammatory markers and may well have positive blood cultures. In very severe cases they may be systemically unwell.

Imaging

Plain film

All patients will have these. Bony changes such as lysis tend to not be visible until late on. In some joints (elbow and ankle) a joint effusion will be visible.

Further imaging

Before any further imaging is undertaken the patient should be reassessed. If the diagnosis based upon the clinical and radiographic findings is definitely of a septic arthritis then the patient should go straight to theatre for a washout that will both confirm the diagnosis and treat the patient.

Ultrasound

This can be used to confirm the presence of an effusion and where appropriate be used to guide joint aspiration.

MRI (Fig. 19.10)

This is reserved for difficult cases where the diagnosis remains in doubt or where there is concern for widespread infection and collections.

Information for the radiologist

- The patient's inflammatory markers, immune status, and clotting status.
- In addition, have they any predisposing clinical condition?
- Finally what is the orthopaedic plan? No intervention should be performed by radiology without appropriate senior discussion with the on-call orthopaedic team.

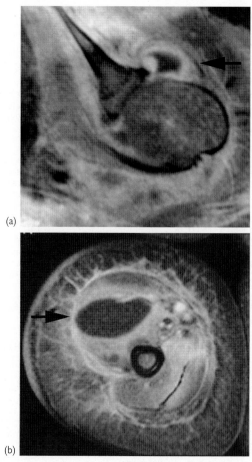

Fig. 19.10 A 9-month-old child with swollen and painful right arm. a) T1 gadolinium axial image at the level of the shoulder joint. The arrow points to pus within the joint consistent with septic arthritis. b) Axial gadolinium image at the level of the mid arm showing further pus within the soft tissues.

Swollen diabetic foot

This is a relatively common and potentially very difficult clinical scenario to deal with. The 3 main areas of concern are:

- Infection.
- Trauma.
- Charcot arthropathy.

The problem is that with severe diabetes the patient may well have an insensate foot that renders clinical examination of little use. Therefore it is essential to take a very careful history and to not be misled by the lack of painful response.

Clinical presentation

All of these conditions will present with a red, swollen foot. The key to differentiating these is the combination of the history, laboratory, and radiological tests. It is also very important to be aware that relatively trivial trauma can cause devastating injuries in the insensate diabetic foot.

Imaging

Plain film (Fig. 19.11)

- These remain the key frontline investigation. In trauma they will demonstrate any injury as well as act as a baseline for follow-up.
- Charcot feet show evidence of advanced OA with destruction, disorganization, debris, dislocation, distention, and increased density. In an acute Charcot foot there will be swelling, bone resorption, and effusions.
- In infection there will be osteolysis, soft tissue swelling, and periosteal reactions.

CT

This is useful for demonstration of the bony anatomy, particularly where there is suspicion for a fracture.

MRI

This is used for assessment of infection and the acute Charcot foot. Both will show similar changes with inflammation, effusions, and bone oedema. However on post-contrast sequences there may well be soft tissue or intra-osseous abscesses in infection. Where there are no collections the MRI findings should be taken in conjunction with laboratory tests to distinguish between these 2 clinical conditions.

Information for the radiologist

Inflammatory markers.

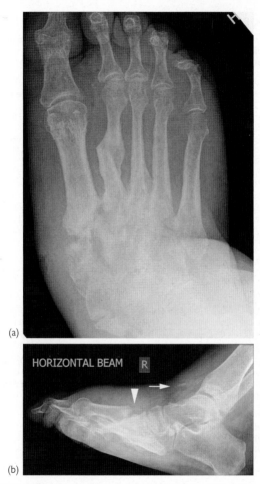

(a)

(b)

Fig. 19.11 A 55-year-old diabetic presented with a painless, swollen foot after tripping over his dog. a) A dorsiplantar radiograph showing marked abnormality to the midfoot. The lateral (b) shows that this is in fact a dislocation across the midfoot (arrowhead). The vascular calcification (arrow) is a classical finding in diabetics.

Loose (painful) joint replacement

The vast majority of joint replacements last for many years, without any problems. In a small percentage they loosen either secondary to infection or loosening of the prosthesis within the cement mantle.

Clinical presentation

Patients presenting with a painful joint after a prosthesis can be divided into 2 groups.

- Early presentation: within 18 months. These can be considered to be infected until proven otherwise.
- Late presentation: after 18 months. These can either be loosening or infection. The longer the prosthesis has been *in situ* the less likely infection is likely to be the cause.

Imaging

Plain film (Fig. 19.12)

All patients get radiographs as part of their follow-up. Both infection and loosening show up as lysis of the cement at the bone–cement interface. Infection tends to cause rapid changes whereas those of aseptic loosening are more gradual.

Ultrasound

This can be used to demonstrate joint effusions and collections. In addition it can used to guide needle aspiration where indicated.

CT/MRI

Both CT and MRI can be used to gain further information regarding the bony and soft tissue anatomy. Unfortunately the metalwork can significantly degrade the image quality and therefore these are limited to specific cases.

Fluoroscopy

Surgeons will usually require confirmation of infection prior to intervening. Fluoroscopy is a good technique to obtain a sample as not only can it be used to guide in the needle but also the images captured are solid evidence of where the sample was obtained.

Information for the radiologist

- When was the prosthesis put in?
- What are the patient's inflammatory markers?
- What is the operative plan?

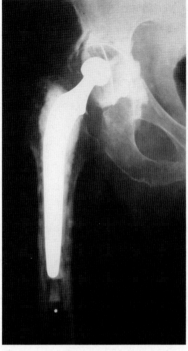

Fig. 19.12 AP radiograph of right hip replacement showing patchy cement lysis of the right femoral component consistent with infection.

Primary bone tumours

Malignant primary bone tumours are a varied group of neoplasms. They account for only 2/1000 cancers diagnosed and are predominantly seen in children or adults >55 years. They arise from the various elements of bone: osteoid (osteosarcoma), cartilage (chondrosarcoma), and neural elements (Ewing's sarcoma).

Clinical presentation

- The age of presentation is the key to the differential diagnosis.
- Pain is the commonest presentation.
- Weight loss or malaise.
- Fever of unknown origin.
- Swelling at the site of pain.
- Pathological fractures.

Imaging

Plain film (Fig. 19.13)

- This is the initial imaging modality of choice.
- 2 films are taken in perpendicular planes.
- 1 of these views needs to show the whole length of the bone.
- The following features are important:
  - Single or multiple.
  - The site of the lesion (epiphyseal, metaphyseal, or diaphyseal).
  - The margins of the lesion (well defined or ill defined).
  - Bony expansion and breach of cortex.
  - Presence of calcification in the lesion or surrounding the lesion.
  - Periosteal reaction.
- A chest radiograph is indicated to exclude metastases.

CT

- This is usually only used to stage the chest.
- Where necessary CT can be used to assess calcification of the lesion.

MRI

- This is used for local staging to assess the full extent of the lesion, which compartments it has breached and whether local neurovascular bundles are involved.
- Standard protocols include T1, fat saturated T2 sequences, and post-contrast T1 images in orthogonal planes.

Scintigraphy

A bone scan is indicated to look for bony metastases.

Information for the radiologist

- Age and presenting symptoms.
- History of malignancy.
- Biochemical markers including parathormone levels if suspicion of hyperparathyroidism or renal failure.
- Tumour markers.

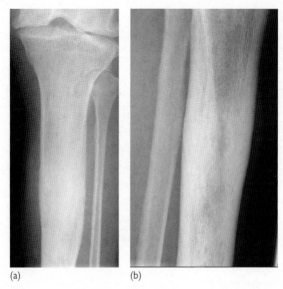

(a) (b)

Fig. 19.13 A 67-year-old male presented with knee pain. a) AP and b) lateral radiographs of the proximal tibia show an area of ill-defined sclerosis with periosteal reaction. This proved to be late onset osteosarcoma of the tibia.

Bone metastases

Bony metastases are common. They may be either osteolytic (bone destroying) or osteosclerotic (bone forming). Primary malignancies produce different types of metastases (see Table 19.3) with osteolytic ones the most common.

Table 19.3 Common malignancies and type of bone metastases

Name	Meaning
Lung	Usually osteolytic
Breast	Either osteolytic or osteosclerotic
Colorectal	Osteolytic
Prostate	Osteosclerotic
Renal cell carcinoma	Osteolytic with expansion
Upper GI cancers	Osteolytic
Gynaecological	Usually osteolytic

Clinical presentation
- Non-specific pain.
- Pyrexia.
- Fractures of the involved bones.

Imaging
Plain film (Fig. 19.14)
- Radiography is the usual first-line investigation.
- Multiple myeloma should always be considered in the differential diagnosis.
- Lytic bone lesions may only cause a subtle discontinuity of the trabeculae. Lung is the most common primary.
- Sclerotic metastases show up as either a generalized bone density increase or as discrete deposits. In men the commonest primary is prostate and in women it is breast.
- Long-bone fractures with irregular and patchy bone texture should raise the suspicion of a metastasis.
- Femoral deposits need prompt recognition, as they can be prophylactically fixed with an intramedullary nail.

CT
- CT is has a high sensitivity for metastatic deposits.
- CT shows metastases best bone windows.
- Definitive diagnosis can be made by a CT-guided biopsy.

Bone scan
- Bone scintigraphy is very good at demonstrating the full extent of bony metastatic spread.

- It shows areas of high bone turnover. Therefore sclerotic metastases may be poorly demonstrated.

MRI

MRI is reserved for problem solving, e.g. differentiating between vertebral body collapse secondary to osteoporosis or metastasis.

PET-CT

- PET is both a functional and anatomical imaging method that can identify metastatic deposits by their glucose uptake.
- PET has a high sensitivity and specificity for identifying bony metastasis and is used after discussion at the MDT.

Information for the radiologist

- Area of the pain.
- Oncological history.
- Tumour markers and calcium levels.

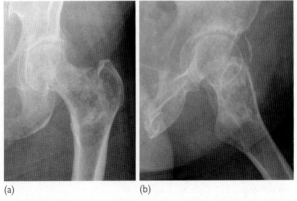

(a)   (b)

Fig. 19.14 A 70-year-old patient presented unable to weight bear after a minor fall. a) AP and b) lateral radiographs show an ill-defined lytic/sclerotic lesion in the intertrochanteric region with a break in the superior cortex. The appearances are consistent with a pathological fracture through a metastasis.

Myeloma

Myeloma is a malignancy characterized by monoclonal proliferation of malignant plasma cells. It is the most common primary malignant neoplasm in adults and commonly occurs in the 5th–8th decades.

- It occurs in 2 forms:
  - Disseminated (more common).
  - Solitary.
- This represents the early stages of multiple myeloma and precedes the disease by 1–20 years.
- Occurs most commonly in the thoracolumbar spine >pelvis >ribs >sternum.

Clinical presentation

Bone destruction

This can lead to:
- Vertebral collapse.
- Hypercalcaemia.

Bone marrow infiltration

- Anaemia.
- Neutropenia.
- Thrombocytopenia.
- Renal impairment.

Imaging

Plain film

Due to the multicentricity of the disease process, a skeletal survey is required to ensure that no regions of disease have been missed.

- Diffuse permeative lesion (can mimic sarcoma or lymphoma).
- Widespread osteolytic lesions with a punched-out appearance and endosteal scalloping.
- Expansile osteolytic lesions (ballooning) in ribs, pelvis, long bones.
- A soft tissue mass may be identified adjacent to the area of bone destruction.

Bone scintigraphy

Myeloma is one of the lesions that is not characteristically 'hot' on a bone scan, therefore plain films are commonly used for the skeletal survey.

CT (Fig. 19.15)

- Acute myeloma: Swiss-cheese pattern, with multiple 'holes' in the bone.
- Chronic myeloma: dense, thick, bony struts.

MRI

MR imaging allows characterization of the bone lesions and any associated soft tissue components.

- T1-weighted: multiple focal hypointense area.
- T2-weighted: corresponding hyperintense regions.
- Characteristic 'mini-brain' appearance.

Information for the radiologist
- Plasma electrophoresis/biochemistry results.
- Site of patient's symptoms.
- History of previous solitary plasmacytoma.

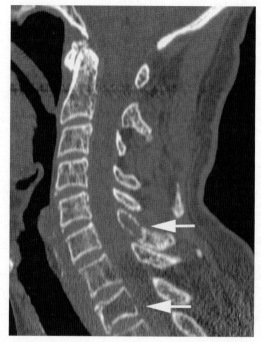

Fig. 19.15 Sagittal CT reformat of the cervical spine demonstrating lytic lesions in the posterior elements of C6 and the body of T1 (arrows) consistent with multiple myeloma.

Benign bone lesions

The most common metaphyseal and epiphyseal benign bone lesions are simple bone cysts, giant cell tumours, and aneurysmal bone cysts.

Clinical presentation

- Asymptomatic.
- History of minor trauma that is unrelated to the condition.
- May present with a pathological fracture.

Imaging

Plain film (Fig. 19.16)

Simple bone cyst
- Skeletally immature patients (epiphyseal fusion has not yet taken place).
- This is the diagnostic modality of choice.
- Simple bone cysts are usually well circumscribed with a single cyst and expansion of the bone. They are commonly seen in the humeral head.
- Pathological fractures through them are common with the 'fallen fragment' sign, a fragment of bone seen within the cyst that has fractured.

Aneurysmal bone cyst (ABC)
- Skeletally immature patients (epiphyseal fusion has not yet taken place).
- An expanded lesion in the bone with multiple cystic areas.
- ABCs do not extend to the joint surface.
- Pathological fractures occur but they do not show the fallen fragment sign.

Giant cell tumour (GCT)
- GCTs are seen in skeletally mature patients.
- This tumour is a multicystic expansile lucent lesion.
- GCTs extend to the joint surface.

CT

CT is used to characterize the fractures in the tumours.

MRI

MRI is used to demonstrate the full extent of these lesions as well as the characteristics of their contents.

Information for the radiologist

- Clinical presentation.
- Patient's age.
- Inflammatory markers.

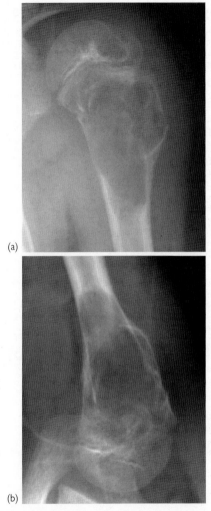

Fig. 19.16 a) AP and b) axial shoulder radiographs taken after patient complained of pain in their shoulder after a fall. These demonstrate a well-defined lucent lesion in the proximal humerus. There is a clear zone of transition. There is a break in the lateral cortex. The appearances are typical of a fracture through a unicameral bone cyst.

Diaphyseal benign bone tumours

Benign bone lesions are relatively uncommon. There are only 3 benign bone lesions that occur in the diaphysis: the fibrous cortical defect (of no clinical concern), fibrous dysplasia (seen in children and resulting in mild deformity of bone), and osteoid osteoma (painful condition affecting children).

Clinical presentation

- Fibrous cortical defects and fibrous dysplasia are usually asymptomatic.
- Non-specific pain. In the case of osteoid osteoma, children get night pain relieved by NSAIDs.
- Fractures of the involved bones.

Imaging

Plain film (Fig. 19.17a)

- Plain radiographs are the modality of choice.
- A fibrous cortical defect is a lytic lesion adjacent to the cortex that disappears after fusion of the growth plate.
- Fibrous dysplasia is a lytic bone lesion with well-defined margins and a 'ground glass' matrix.
- Osteoid osteoma is a bone-forming tumour that presents as a thickened area of cortex in a long bone although vertebral body osteomas are also known.

CT

- CT has a high sensitivity for osteoid osteoma and is the modality of choice to confirm the diagnosis.
- CT shows a thick cortex with a lucent area in the centre.
- Definitive diagnosis is often made by a CT-guided biopsy and is used to guide therapy.

Bone scintigraphy

Osteoid osteomas have high bone turnover and will show as a focus of high uptake.

MRI (Fig. 19.17b)

MRI is reserved for difficult atypical cases.

Information for the radiologist

- Area of the pain.
- Relevant history.
- Relevant biochemical results including tumour markers and calcium levels.

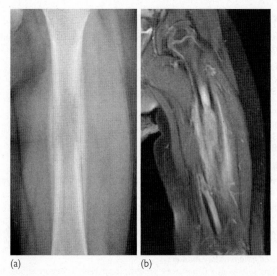

(a)   (b)

Fig. 19.17 An 8-year-old patient presented with a 2-month history of left thigh pain. a) AP radiograph shows mid diaphyseal lesion with chronic perosteal reaction and medullary lysis. b) T1FS coronal MRI shows extensive inflammation associated with this but no soft tissue mass. The appearances are consistent with eosinophic granuloma.

Sclerotic bone lesions

The underlying cause for these range from congenital abnormalities through to malignant secondaries.

Benign causes

- Osteoid osteoma.
- Bone island.
- Chondroid lesion.
- Paget's disease.
- Infection.
- Sequestrum.
- Bone infarct.

Clinical presentation

This is important as presentation can help to differentiate the underlying cause.

Incidental finding

In an otherwise well patient this is an essentially reassuring scenario and would imply that may it well be long-standing in nature. This does not exclude aggressive lesions.

Raised inflammatory markers

In this setting an inflammatory process, most likely infection, should be actively investigated as obviously if this is the cause then it is treatable.

Pain

The type of pain can be very helpful as ostoid osteomas classically present with night pain that is relieved by NSAIDs. Night pain is, as a rule, a worrying symptom and will warrant a full work-up for an aggressive aetiology.

Imaging

Plain film

These remain the mainstay for initial investigation and usually will provide the diagnosis. Key findings are the transition zone, the age of the patient, and the location of the lesion. Lesions with ill-defined margins tend to be aggressive whereas a well-demarcated margin with a sclerotic edge is reassuring.

CT (Fig. 19.18)

This is good for looking at the bony anatomy and the zone of transition. CT will confirm the diagnosis of osteoid osteoma by confirming its intra-cortical location. In cases of infection it will demonstrate sequestra (dead pieces of bone) that can act as nutrient reservoirs for bugs.

MRI

This is good for demonstrating the soft tissue elements of a lesion as well as involvement of joints and local neurovascular bundles. In cases of infection this will show the full extent of any osteomyelitis as well as any abscesses.

Information for the radiologist

- Does the patient have a known primary tumour?
- Is the lesion painful and if so when.

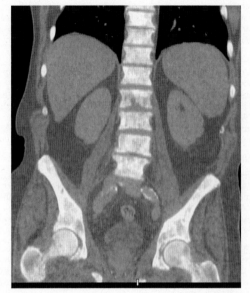

Fig. 19.18 Coronal CT reformation of the pelvis and lumbar spine showing widespread sclerotic lesions consistent with disseminated prostate metastases.

Paget's disease

This is a condition where there is a localized increase in size and numbers of osteoclasts leading to an increased rate of osteolysis. This is followed by a compensatory increase in osteoblasts causing accelerated bone deposition. This combination of factors results in the classical Pagetic appearance with a larger, chaotic and sclerotic bone. In early stages areas of ostolysis will be seen, classically in the skull—osteoporosis circumscripta.

Clinical presentation

- This rarely occurs in patients <40 years of age. The majority of patients are asymptomatic and it is a purely coincidental finding.
- Symptomatic patients complain of bone pain, headache, hearing-loss, and hip pain. As Pagetic bone loses its flexibility pathological fractures are well described.
- Sarcomatous change in osteosaroma can occur in 1% of patients as a complication of Paget's disease.

Imaging

Plain film (Fig. 19.19)

These are the mainstay for diagnosis and follow-up of Paget's disease. This classically demonstrates and enlarged, sclerotic bone with a prominent trabecular pattern.

Incremental stress fractures are well seen on these and develop on the convex sides of long bones.

Bone scintigraphy

Paget's shows a classical whole bone intense activity that is usually diagnostic from the far end of the reporting room. Exceptions to this are when there is sarcomatous change or in osteoporosis circumscripta where there will be areas of lower uptake.

CT and MRI

These are good at demonstrating the full extent of the bony involvement. They are, however, reserved for difficult cases where the diagnosis is in doubt or where there has been sarcomatous change to assess the extent of the tumour.

Information for the radiologist

What are the patient's symptoms and has there been any recent change in these?

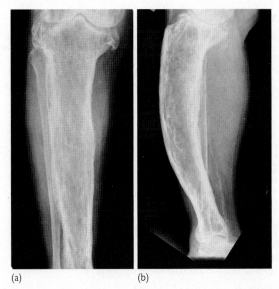

(a)   (b)

Fig. 19.19 a) AP radiograph of tibia showing the classical enlarged bone with prominent sclerotic trabeculae. b) Image shows the marked bowing of the tibia.

Avascular necrosis

Avascular necrosis (AVN), also known as osteonecrosis, is the cellular death of bone secondary to interruption of its blood supply. It affects bones with a single terminal blood supply and is most commonly seen in the epiphyses of long bones, e.g. the femoral head.

Causes of avascular necrosis

- Idiopathic.
- Trauma.
- Steroids.
- Alcohol.
- Caisson disease.
- Haemoglobinopathies.
- Connective tissue disorders.
- Hyperlipidaemia.
- Renal transplant.
- Gaucher's disease.
- Radiotherapy.
- Bisphosphonates (osteonecrosis of mandible).

Clinical presentation

AVN may be asymptomatic and an incidental finding. The commonest presenting feature is pain followed by decreased range of movement.

Imaging

Plain film (Fig. 19.20)

Plain radiographs are often normal. Early radiographic findings are subtle changes in bone density. Features of advanced disease include suchondral lucencies, collapse of the articular surface, and deformity. The joint space is preserved until late in the disease.

MRI

This is the most sensitive modality for the detection of AVN. The earliest sign is decreased contrast enhancement in areas of compromised blood supply. Bone marrow oedema best seen on T1-weighted images is an early non-specific sign.

Later, after the onset of osseous repair the classical double line sign may be demonstrated in 80% of cases on T2-weighted sequences. This sign describes an inner hyperintense line (hyperaemic granulation tissue) and an outer hypointense line (chemical shift artifact). This sign is considered pathognomonic of the AVN.

Nuclear medicine

While MRI is the modality of choice in suspected AVN, bone scintigraphy and SPECT may be used in the diagnostic work-up of a patient with bone pain. The main feature described is a cold spot representing the area of ischaemia which may have a surrounding area of increased signal.

Information for the radiologist

The site of pain, duration of symptoms, and any risk factors for AVN.

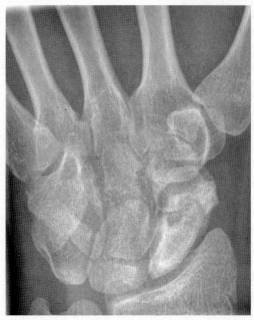

Fig. 19.20 Scaphoid radiograph showing a scaphoid non-union. The proximal pole of the scaphoid is more sclerotic than any of the carpal bones consistent with AVN.

Osteoporosis

Reduced bone mass due to equal reduction in both osteoid (matrix) and hydroxyapatite (mineral) content. The proportion of mineralization remains the same and is normal. It may be primary (age related) or secondary to another condition.

Secondary causes include:
- Malabsorption (e.g. coeliac/Crohn's).
- Renal failure.
- Hyperparathyroidism.
- Drugs (e.g. steroids, heparin, anticonvulsants).
- Oophorectomy (hypogonadism).
- Cushing's syndrome.
- Acromegaly.
- Rheumatological disease.
- Haematological disease.

Clinical presentation

Presentation is usually with osteoporotic fractures or through screening in those with risk factors (listed). Common sites for fracture are the distal radius, femoral neck, wedge fractures of thoracic and lumbar vertebrae. All these occur with minimal trauma, which should alert the clinician to the underlying cause.

Risk factors

- Increasing age.
- Female sex.
- Smoking.
- Excess alcohol.
- Lack of exercise.
- Early menopause.
- Low body mass index.
- Family history.

Imaging

Plain film

Diffuse osteopenia with cortical thinning may be present, although there has to be significant bone loss before the changes become radiographically apparent. This can make early disease detection difficult. Fractures of the sites listed previously with resulting kyphosis of the thoracic and lumbar spine may be identified.

Dual energy X-ray absorptiometry (DEXA)

This is the most accurate and widely available technique. Multiple sites are assessed and a standard deviation from the mean of a young adult (T-score) is obtained. The World Health Organization definitions are:[1]
- Normal: T >1.
- Osteopenia: T <−1 to >−2.5.
- Osteoporosis: T <−2.5.

MRI/CT/NM: none of these are routinely used in the diagnosis of osteoporosis.

Information for the radiologist

Any relevant risk factors or possible primary causes. Suspicion due to previous characteristic fractures.

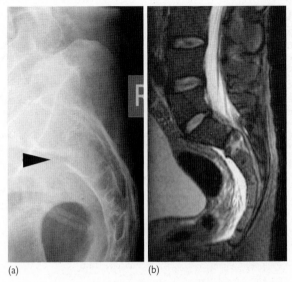

(a)   (b)

Fig. 19.21 A 25-year-old alcoholic who fell down onto his bottom. a) Image shows a fracture through the sacrum. b) A STIR sagittal MRI confirming the extent of this fracture. This is an unusual injury in such a young person and is consistent with severe osteoporosis secondary to alcohol abuse.

Reference

1 World Health Organization. Assessment of Fracture Risk and its Application to Screening for Postmenopausal Osteoporosis. WHO Technical Report Series 843. Geneva: World Health Organization, 1994.

Osteomalacia

Abnormality of the bones due to reduced bone mineralization that occurs during adulthood. Failure of mineralization in children results in rickets. Histology shows a reduction in hydroxyapatite but normal osteoid matrix content.

Clinical presentation

Presents with bone pain, non-specific aches, fractures, and proximal muscle weakness. A waddling gait and confirmation of proximal muscle weakness is found on examination. Blood tests are not diagnostic and vary during disease stages. They can include low phosphate, low calcium, low vitamin D, raised alkaline phosphatase, and raised parathyroid hormone.

Causes

- Vitamin D deficiency:
  - Reduced sunlight exposure
  - Low oral intake
  - Malabsorption
  - Liver disease
- Vitamin D-dependent rickets (hereditary)
- Multiple myeloma
- Renal disease:
  - Chronic renal failure
  - Dialysis related bone disease
  - Renal tubular acidosis
  - Fanconi's syndrome
- X-linked phosphataemia rickets (hereditary)
- Anticonvulsants

Imaging

Plain film (Fig. 19.22)

Looser's zone (pseudofractures) are radiolucent lines with sclerotic margins that extend from the cortex. These are most commonly found in the medial femoral neck, axillary border of scapula, ribs, and pubic rami. In more severe disease a complete pathological fracture may occur. Patients usually have coarsening of the trabeculae, however some may have generalized osteopenia.

MRI/CT

These can be used to identify early radiographically occult fractures. This is usually when there is a high index of clinical suspicion but no radiographic abnormality present. They also have a role where the radiographic findings are inconclusive.

Nuclear medicine

Bone scan shows diffusely increased uptake with no evidence of renal excretion which is termed a 'superscan' appearance. This can also be used to confirm fractures.

Information for the radiologist

Clinical history and serological tests may help. Conveying a suspicion of osteomalacia is essential to diagnose the subtle plain film changes.

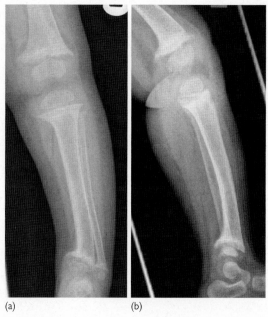

(a)   (b)

Fig. 19.22 Images a) and b) demonstrate the pathognomonic appearances of rickets with splaying and fraying of the metaphyses.

Trauma

Head trauma

It is now well recognized that the prompt recognition of intracranial injuries and their treatment has a significant impact upon these patients' morbidity and mortality. This has led to the development of the NICE head injury guidelines.[1]

Clinical presentation

Patients with any of the following presentations, post head injury, have a risk of significant head injury:

- GCS <13.
- GCS <15 2 hours after the accident.
- Suspected open, depressed, or basal skull fracture.
- Post-traumatic seizure.
- >1 episode of vomiting in adults and >3 in children.
- Coagulopathy.
- Focal neurological deficit.

Imaging

Plain film

These now have very little use in this scenario except where the demonstration of a fracture will alter management, e.g. non-accidental injury.

CT (Fig. 20.1)

This is indicated for all of the earlier listed scenarios as soon as is possible in the receiving hospital. The aim of this is to identify treatable intracranial bleeds that will require prompt intervention. These will also act as baseline scans for comparison later if the patient deteriorates and has a follow-up scan.

Where there is evidence significant head trauma discussion about whether the cervical spine should be imaged at the same time.

MRI

There are no clear guidelines for the use of MRI in head injuries. It clearly demonstrates white matter injuries very well and at present is used in difficult cases after senior discussion.

Information for the radiologist

A clear history of the injury, mechanism, and clinical course of the patient post injury, listing any of the earlier listed justifications for imaging.

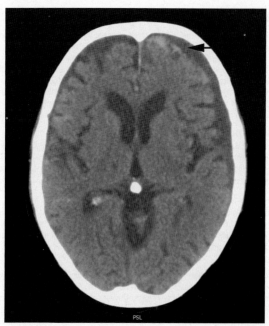

Fig. 20.1 An 85-year-old man admitted with reduced level of consciousness after falling over. The arrow points to an acute subdural bleed (white area). The fluid in the subdural space would indicate previous bleeds making this an acute on chronic subdural haemorrhage.

Reference

1 NICE. *Head Injury. NICE clinical guideline 5*. London: NICE, 2007.

Facial trauma

Facial trauma used to be a very common problem in emergency departments. The mandatory use of seatbelts in combination with the more recent introduction of airbags and crumple zones has massively reduced these.

The facial bones act as the head's own crumple zone and so it is possible to have massive facial injuries with relatively little injury to the brain.

However, the face has a very rich blood supply making immediate treatment of these challenging. The long-term cosmetic implications in the modern era where image is so highly valued should not be underestimated.

Clinical presentation

By definition these are the result of trauma. This is usually by a blunt mechanism such as a fist, although penetrating injuries do occur. The more imaginative of the latter often then find themselves reported in the gutter press.

Imaging

This used to be by plain radiography although these are notoriously difficult to interpret. They can, however, be used as a screening tool as significant fluid with the sinuses has a good predictive value for fractures in the trauma setting.

CT

With the introduction of multislice CT technology this is the imaging modality of choice for assessment of facial trauma. A volumetric acquisition is made and then high quality reformations in any plane can be produced as well as 3D models to guide the surgeon (Fig. 20.2).

The true extent of facial injuries is only now really being appreciated with the well-established classifications being revisited and updated. For example, the pterygoid plates could never be visualized by plain radiography but are beautifully seen on CT. For the reporting radiologist they are key landmarks as fractures of these immediately equate to a LeFort type injury.

Information for the radiologist

• Trauma mechanism.
• Any known previous injuries.

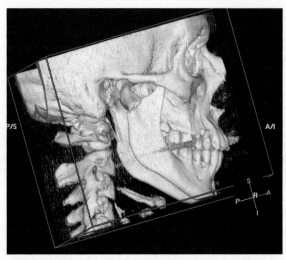

Fig. 20.2 3D CT reconstruction demonstrating right mandibular condyle fracture with dislocation of the temporomandibular joint.

Spinal trauma

This is common in polytrauma and there may be multiple injuries. The unconscious patient can be particularly challenging to investigate. Early diagnosis reduces the risk of potentially devastating neurological sequelae.

Cervical spine injury can lead to cervical cord injury with resultant respiratory arrest. Thoracolumbar injuries can lead to paralysis and are frequently overlooked.

Clinical presentation

Pain at the site of injury or neurological disturbance. Look for bruising, swelling, deformity, and localized spinal tenderness. A full neurological assessment should be documented, including perianal sensation, anal sphincter tone, and evidence of urinary retention. The Canadian C-spine rules can be applied to 'clear' low-risk patients of cervical spine injury on clinical grounds whilst the remainder should proceed to imaging.[1]

Imaging

Plain film

Standard views are lateral, AP, and an open mouth view of C1/C2 if the C-spine is imaged. C-spine radiographs should include the C7/T1 junction.

Indicators of injury include visible fracture lines, bone fragments, soft tissue swelling, reduced vertebral body height, facet joint malalignment, and widened interspinous distance.

Flexion/extension views: not suitable in the acute setting and performed only with extreme caution by an experienced clinician. Can reveal occult ligamentous injuries.

CT

This is highly sensitive for bone injury. Indicated if radiographs are inadequate, a fracture is seen on plain film, or if clinical findings are discordant with radiographic findings. However, a normal CT does not exclude ligamentous injury.

MRI

This is superior to CT and radiography in demonstrating soft tissue injuries such as ligamentous disruption, cord compression, or epidural haemorrhage. Patients with neurological compromise usually proceed to MRI.

Information for the radiologist

• Timing and mode of injury, site of pain or tenderness.
• Neurological findings including which side and the neurological level.

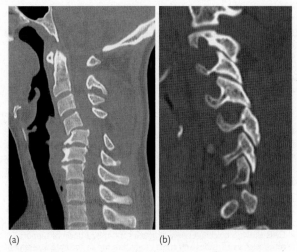

(a)   (b)

Fig. 20.3 A 45-year-old male who had crashed his motor-cycle into a wall at 80mph. a) A mid-line sagittal CT reformation of the cervical spine showing an angular kyphosis at C4/5 with massive widening of the interlaminar space posteriorly consistent with a flexion injury. b) A parasagittal reformation showing the perched facet at C4/5.

Reference

1 Stiell IG, Wells GA, Vandemheen KL, et al. The Canadian C-Spine rule study for alert and stable trauma patients. JAMA 2001; **286**:1841–8.

Thoracic trauma

Chest trauma can be due to blunt or penetrating injury. The spectrum of potential injuries is wide but remember to check:

- A: airway.
- A: aorta.
- B: bones.
- C: cardiac.
- D: diaphragm.
- E: (o)esophagus.

Clinical presentation

Depend on the location and type of injury, but acute dyspnoea, pallor, shock, cold extremities, tenderness over chest wall are typical in severe cases. Many cases will be associated with severe injury to other systems.

Imaging

Plain film

- Still has a role in poly trauma but should not delay resuscitation or movement of patient to CT scanner.
- CXR allows a quick overview of injuries and the position of support tubes such as ET tubes and chest drains, but for an accurate assessment of injuries CT is required.
- Has a high negative predictive value for aortic injury if normal but have high level of suspicion if aortic arch not clearly seen.

CT (Fig. 20.4)

- CT of the chest should be part of radiological assessment in all cases of severe polytrauma.
- Gives accurate assessment of lung, mediastinal, bony, and diaphragmatic injuries.
- A normal, good quality CT has an almost 100% negative predictive value for aortic injury.

Ultrasound

Can be used to look for haemothorax or pneumothorax in experienced hands, but is not as accurate as CT.

MRI

Little role in acute setting, but can be useful in delayed diagnosis of diaphragm rupture.

Angiography

Largely replaced by multislice CT as a diagnostic tool, but developing an ever-increasing role in the treatment of acute vascular injury, including aortic transection.

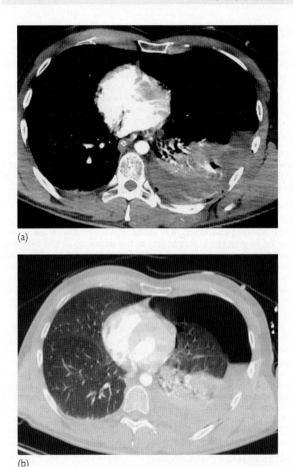

(a)

(b)

Fig. 20.4 Axial CT images from a patient who sustained multiple injuries following a road traffic accident. a) The first CT is viewed on 'mediastinal' windows, showing fluid within the left chest, and active bleeding, seen as contrast dependently within the lower left chest. b) The second CT is the same image viewed on 'lung' windows, showing an associated pneumothorax.

Abdominal trauma

This remains a major cause of morbidity and mortality in the Western world. Perhaps not surprisingly road traffic accidents (RTAs) remain the major cause even with modern safety developments.

Traditional ATLS® (Advanced Trauma Life Support) management relied upon good clinical history taking, examination and basic bedside tests. The exponential improvement in CT technology means that, where available, CT really should be the C in the ABC approach.

Clinical presentation

The presentation can be variable although high-energy mechanisms should raise concern that for an intra-abdominal injury. Obviously direct trauma to the abdomen or lower rib cage carries a very high risk and there should be a very low threshold for imaging these patients.

Imaging

Ultrasound

FAST (focused assessment with sonography for trauma) scans remain popular in emergency departments as the demonstration of free fluid confirms that there is an intra-abdominal injury. Unfortunately ultrasound remains very poor at delineating the injuries themselves and is of little value in assessing bowel trauma.

Ultrasound does, however, retain a role in following-up known injuries, particularly in children where dose is an issue.

CT (Fig. 20.5)

It is now well recognized that anyone with presenting with injuries to 2 or more major body parts should have a Pan-Scan (vertex to symphysis). This is because these patients often have multiple injuries some of which can be very difficult to locate surgically.

Traditional teaching is that no haemodynamically unstable patient should go for a CT scan. Once again the speed of modern scanners means that patients spend very little time in the scan room. Indeed the rapid and accurate identification of life-threatening injuries is unsurpassed by any other approach.

Once the scan is done and all the injuries identified then a management plan for the patient for the remainder of his hospital stay can be drawn up.

Information for the radiologist

- Mechanism of injury.
- Known injuries.
- Haemodynamic status.

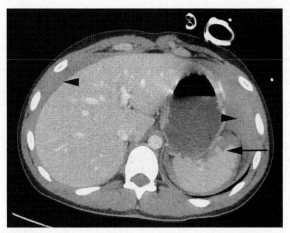

Fig. 20.5 Trauma. A 35-year-old female who had fallen off her horse. Axial CT showing active bleeding from the spleen (arrow) and intra-abdominal free blood (arrowheads).

Pelvic fractures

Pelvic fractures are associated with high-energy injuries (in the UK either RTAs or falls from a height). The incidence of pelvic fractures in patients with blunt trauma is approximately 10%. The pelvis is an extremely resilient skeletal structure whose integrity is maintained by extremely strong ligaments and powerful muscles.

Hence, any trauma to the pelvis has a high risk of injury to the soft tissues, abdominal organs, and spine. The most important association is with active bleeding.

Clinical presentation

The main mechanisms of injury occur through 3 vectors:

- AP compression: this is the commonest type of injury characterized by pubic diastasis ± sacroiliac (SI) joint disruption. AP compression can result in an increase in the volume of the pelvis putting the patient at risk of exsanguination.
- Lateral compression: the hallmark of lateral compression fractures is the fracture of the pubic rami with sacral buckle fractures. This is associated with intra-abdominal and intra-pelvic injuries but is less likely to have major pelvic haemorrhage.
- Vertical shear injuries occur due to a vertical force, often from the femur. There are vertical fractures of the pubic rami and SI joints with ligamentous disruption and hemi-pelvic displacement.

Imaging

Plain film

The AP pelvis film allows the initial assessment of the pelvic bones and their alignment (Fig. 20.6).

CT

- CT is the modality of choice for assessment of pelvic injuries, as not only does it give detailed analysis of the fractures but it demonstrates the associated soft tissue injuries.
- The most important finding is of active bleeding.

MRI

MRI can help in identifying occult fractures of the pelvis and hips.

Information for the radiologist

- Mechanism of injury.
- The haemodynamic status of the patient.

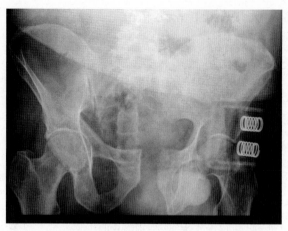

Fig. 20.6 A 65-year-old male admitted after frontal impact in an RTA. AP pelvic radiograph which demonstrates disruption to the pubic symphysis and external rotation of the left hemi-pelvis. This is consistent with an AP compression injury (open book).

Shoulder trauma

Shoulder trauma presents with a variety of fracture/dislocation patterns. Usually it is the result of a fall onto an awkwardly held arm.

Clinical presentation

Patients with a fracture can usually get the arm into a semi-comfortable position compared to a dislocation, which is exceptionally painful no matter what they do.

Imaging

Plain film

Most shoulder injuries can be diagnosed with conventional radiography.

Clavicular fracture

These commonly occur at the junction between the middle and outer thirds. There may be displacement and fragment overlap.

Acromio-clavicular (AC) joint subluxation/dislocation (Fig. 20.7)

Seen as widening and vertical separation of the AC joint space. Comparison or weight-bearing views of both shoulders can be helpful.

Anterior dislocation (commonest)

This is characterized by subcoracoid position of the humeral head on the AP view. The dislocation is often more obvious in a scapular 'Y' view, where the humeral head lies anterior to the 'Y.' In the axillary view, the 'golf ball' (i.e. humeral head) falls anterior to the 'tee' (i.e. glenoid).

Posterior dislocation (2%)

The AP view may show medial rotation of the humeral head, resembling a light bulb. The scapular 'Y' view reveals the humeral head behind the glenoid (the centre of the 'Y'). In an axillary view, the 'golf ball' falls posteriorly off the 'tee'.

Inferior dislocation (rare)

The patient presents with arm held abducted above the head. The AP view may show the arm raised over the head with the humeral head inferior to the glenoid.

Humeral neck/head fracture

These are often impacted or oblique fractures. They are classified according to separation of the head, shaft, greater and lesser tuberosities (Neer classification).

CT

Indicated for radiographically occult injuries and for surgical planning of complex fractures.

MRI

This is the investigation of choice for soft tissue, cartilage, and bone marrow assessment.

Information for the radiologist

Does the mechanism match the injury demonstrated?

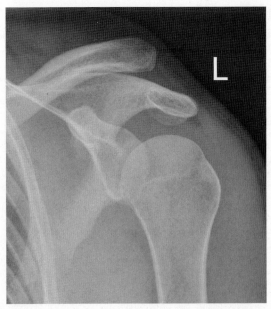

Fig. 20.7 A 30-year-old male who fell off his mountain bike and has presented with a grossly deformed left shoulder joint. The figure shows dislocation of the acromio-clavicular joint.

Elbow trauma

The elbow is a hinge joint comprising the radius, ulna, and humerus. These are at risk when falling onto the outstretched arm.

Clinical presentation

Injuries to the elbow joint can lead to a loss in flexion, extension, or even a locked joint.

Imaging

Plain film

This is the mainstay of trauma imaging for the elbow with CT and MRI limited to complex injuries.

Elbow joint effusion

This is the single most important finding. Fat pads, which lie on the anterior and posterior surfaces of the distal humerus, are not usually visualized. With an elbow joint effusion, they are lifted off the humeral surface and seen on the lateral view as dark grey triangular structures. In trauma, they are associated with fractures even if one is not readily seen (usually an undisplaced radial head or supracondylar fracture).

Anterior humeral line and radiocapitellar line

The anterior humeral line is drawn along the anterior cortex of the distal humerus and should pass through the middle 1/3 of the capitellum. Malalignment indicates the presence of a fracture (e.g. supracondylar or lateral condyle fractures).

The radiocapitellar line demonstrates the congruence between the radial head and the capitellum. The line should be drawn through the proximal radius and should intersect the centre of the capitellum on any view. Malalignment indicates dislocation of the elbow or radial head.

Elbow fractures

There are multiple fracture types with the most common being the radial head/neck and supracondylar humeral fractures.

In paediatric patients, always look for the medial epicondyle as if avulsed it is pulled into the joint and can be difficult to identify.

Elbow dislocation

These are classified according to the direction of dislocation and associated fractures. The most frequent injury is posterolateral dislocation.

Information for the radiologist

Is the joint locked or is there a loss of extension or flexion?

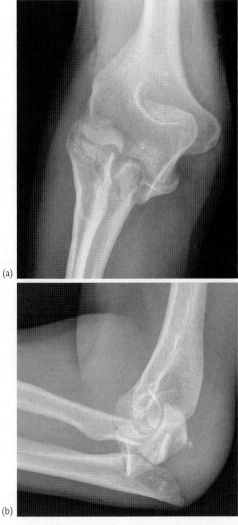

Fig. 20.8 Images a) and b) demonstrate a multisegmental fracture of the elbow with significant displacement of the ulna shaft from the olecranon.

Hand and wrist trauma

Clinical presentation

Patients with a fracture can usually get the arm into a semi-comfortable position compared to a dislocation, which is exceptionally painful no matter what they do.

Imaging

Plain film (Figs. 20.9 and 20.10)

This remains the mainstay for imaging for these areas as most injuries are well demonstrated by plain films. Where the imaging doesn't match the clinical findings then further investigations should be considered.

Distal radial fractures

The classic Colles' fracture consists of a transverse fracture of the distal radius (within 2.5cm of the wrist) with dorsal angulation of the distal fragment. It may be associated with avulsion of the ulnar styloid process.

The less common Smith's fracture refers to volar angulation of the distal radial fragment and is very unstable.

Scaphoid fracture

Specialized scaphoid views should be obtained (AP, lateral, right, and left obliques). The scaphoid most commonly fractures transversely through the waist, but sometimes through the tubercle. Waist fractures are associated with a high incidence of avascular necrosis of the proximal pole due to interruption of its blood supply, which is via the distal pole.

Scaphoid fractures may not be visible on initial radiographs. Snuffbox tenderness without a radiographically visible fracture should be followed up closely with clinical review. Persisting symptoms after 10–14 days require further imaging with either a bone scan or MRI to identify any underlying injury.

Lunate dislocation

This is a rare but often missed injury. The lunate dislocates anteriorly. This may be difficult to appreciate on the AP film, but is more easily seen on the lateral view with the lunate rotated and displaced anteriorly.

Perilunate dislocation

In perilunate dislocation, the lunate remains attached to the radius with the remainder of the carpal bones displaced posteriorly. There is only minimal, if any, rotation of the lunate. This injury is often associated with a scaphoid fracture (trans-scaphoidperilunate dislocation), or fracture of the radial styloid.

Other carpal fractures

Avulsion fracture of the posterior surface of the triquetral may be seen on the lateral view as a small fragment adjacent to the dorsal surface of the bone. It is also possible to fracture any of the other carpal bones, but this tends to be much less common.

Ligament and cartilage injuries

The wrist contains many important ligaments and cartilages that support the carpal bones and which may be injured following trauma. The most commonly injured structures include the scapholunate ligament, triquetrolunate ligament and the triangular fibrocartilage complex. These injuries are best investigated with stress views (to demonstrate carpal instability) or MRI.

Metacarpals and phalanges

These are common fractures. It is important to assess the degree of angulation/displacement to guide further management.

Thumb

Bennet's fracture-dislocation describes fracture of the base of the first metacarpal which extends into the carpometacarpal joint (i.e. it is intra-articular). There is lateral subluxation of the main metacarpal fragment.

A Rolando fracture is a comminuted intra-articular fracture through the base of the 1st metacarpal consisting of 3 distinct fragments; it is typically T- or Y-shaped.

Information for the radiologist

What is the mechanism of injury and does the imaging match the clinical findings?

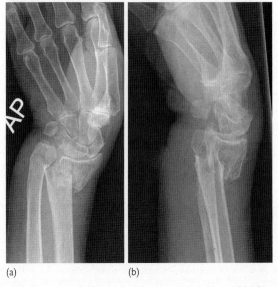

(a)　　　　　　　　(b)

Fig. 20.9 This is a 60-year-old lady who fell over on the ice with a painful deformed wrist. a) AP view showing gross deformity with significant radial translation. b) The lateral confirms significant dorsal translation.

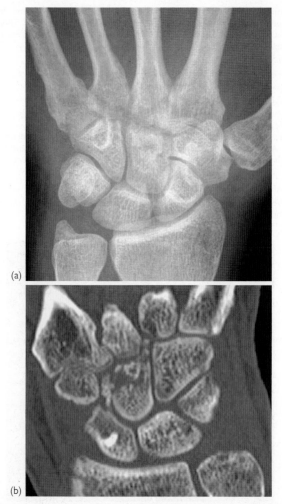

Fig. 20.10 A 20-year-old male with a painful hand after punching a wall. a) The AP radiograph is difficult to interpret but the middle carpometacarpal joint is indistinct as is the distal capitate. b) Coronal CT reformat confirms a multi-segmental fracture of the capitate involving the middle carpometacarpal joint.

Proximal femoral fractures

Lower limb fracture patterns can present in a number of ways, depending on mechanism of injury, age of patient, and underlying bone strength. The femur requires large forces to fracture or dislocate it, except in cases of osteoporosis, tumour, or infection.

Clinical presentation

Fractured neck of femur (NOF)

This is a common injury in the elderly. Patients present with groin pain or pain radiating to the knee following a fall and inability to weight bear. On examination the leg is often shortened and externally rotated.

Intracapsular fractures

Subcapital, cervical, and basal fractures disrupt the blood supply to the femoral head leading to avascular necrosis. These are treated with a hemiarthroplasty.

Extracapsular fractures

Intertrochanteric, basal and subtrochanteric fractures do not disrupt the blood supply and therefore can be treated by fixation, e.g. dynamic hip screw (DHS).

Hip dislocation

These are usually secondary to high-energy trauma in younger patients. They can be divided into anterior, posterior (80%), or central. Fractures of the acetabular margin are a common complication of posterior dislocations.

Imaging

Plain film (Fig. 20.11)

- AP and lateral views are the first line of investigation.
- A fracture line, cortical or trabecular disruption may be identified.

CT

- This should only be used to characterize complex fractures.
- 3D reconstruction views can aid surgical planning.

MRI

This is indicated where there is strong clinical concern for a femoral neck fracture but the radiographs are negative. 2% of all femoral neck fractures are radiographically occult. MRI can assess soft tissues, occult fractures, and underlying bone.

Bone scintigraphy

Where MRI is contraindicated or not available this can be used as an alternative to investigate an occult femoral neck fracture.

Information for the radiologist

- Does the mechanism match the injury?
- Does there remain a strong clinical concern for a femoral neck fracture?

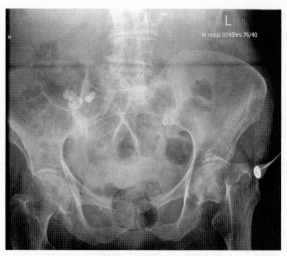

Fig. 20.11 An 85-year-old patient, who was found on the floor with a shortened and externally rotated left leg. Pelvic radiograph demonstrates a multisegmental fracture of the left femoral neck.

Knee injuries

The inherent stability of the knee is dependent on the associated soft tissues:
- Extra-articular ligaments (medial and lateral collateral).
- Intra-articular ligaments (anterior and posterior cruciate).
- Menisci.

Common injuries

Cruciate ligament injury

Injuries to these classically present as an immediate haemarthrosis after injury.
  An avulsion fracture often accompanies a rupture of one of the ligaments.
- Fractures of the tibial spine are a consequence of avulsions of the anterior cruciate ligament.
- Posterior cruciate injuries are associated with an avulsion fracture, posterior to the tibial spines.
- A Segond fracture is a capsular avulsion fracture of the margin of the lateral tibial plateau and is strongly associated with anterior cruciate and meniscal injuries.

Meniscal injuries

These classically present with locking, clicking, and effusion. The latter becomes apparent several hours after the injury.

Collateral ligament injuries

These present after a blow to the knee from the side with associated instability.

Tibial plateau fractures

Significant injuries to the medial and lateral collateral ligaments are often associated with these fractures.
- 80% involve the lateral plateau.
- They may be subtle, but can be identified on radiographs as a depression in the plateau secondary to impaction from the femoral condyle.
- There may be displacement of the tibial margin.

Patella

- Following a direct blow to the patella, comminuted fractures may be seen.
- Osteochondral fractures of the articular surface may occur secondary to patella dislocation. Skyline views or MRI may be required to demonstrate this injury.
- Common sites are: the medial surface of the patella or the lateral femoral condyle.

Imaging

Plain film

AP
- This is good for assessment of the assessment of all 3 bones and their coronal alignment.
- Beware confusing a bipartite patella (characteristic position in the upper outer quadrant) with a fracture.

Lateral
- This view can demonstrate evidence of an effusion or a lipohaemarthrosis (indicated by a fat-fluid level in the effusion).
- A lipohaemarthrosis may be the only plain film sign of an intra-articular fracture.

Oblique or skyline views are indicated if a patellar injury is suspected.

CT
This is commonly used to confirm subtle injuries or for surgical planning in complex cases, e.g. tibial plateau fractures.

MRI
This is the modality of choice for the diagnosis of soft tissues injuries around the knee including; meniscal and ligament sprains and tears.

Information for the radiologist
- The mechanism of injury.
- Surgical plan and anticipated timescale.

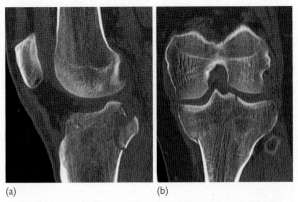

(a)   (b)

Fig. 20.12 A 25-year-old female who was on the receiving end of a 2-footed sliding tackle. a) Sagittal and b) coronal CT reformats showing an intra-articular fracture of the proximal tibia.

Ankle trauma

The ankle is a hinge joint formed by the tibia, talus, and fibula. The joint is weak anteriorly and posteriorly, but reinforced by the medial collateral, lateral collateral, and the interosseous ligaments.

Clinical presentation

Mechanisms of injury occur via:
- Inversion injury (damage to lateral ligaments ± malleolus).
- Eversion injury (this stresses the medial ligament and may avulse the medial malleolus).
- Forced dorsiflexion.

Common fractures

Malleoli
- These fractures are usually obvious, although both views should be inspected carefully, as some are only seen on one view.
- If a fracture is identified then look for a 2nd fracture or a ligamentous injury.

Talus
Osteochondral fractures:
- Small talar dome impaction fractures.
- Often occur during inversion.

Neck of talus:
- These have a high associated risk of avascular necrosis.

Body of talus:
- These have a risk of non-union or subsequent subtalar osteoarthritis if unrecognized.

Imaging

Plain film
These are the main investigation of ankle injuries (if positive Ottawa ankle rules).

AP mortice
- The joint space should be uniform with a smooth surface to the talar dome.
- The space between distal tibia and fibula should not measure >6mm.

Lateral
This should include the calcaneus and the base of 5th metatarsal.

CT
This is used if there is a strong clinical suspicion of a fracture, but the plain films are negative, or if detailed reconstructions are required for surgical planning.

MRI
This is indicated for significant ligamentous, cartilage, osteochondral, and soft tissue injuries.

Classification

The Weber–AO classification system is the most commonly used ankle fracture classification system. This refers to injuries to the lateral malleolus:

- Type A: fracture below the ankle joint.
- Type B: fracture at the level of the joint.
- Type C: fracture above joint level, which tears the syndesmotic ligaments.

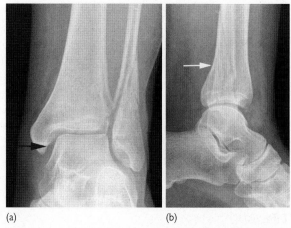

(a)   (b)

Fig. 20.13 A 25-year-old fell awkwardly whilst playing football. a) AP and b) lateral radiographs demonstrate a multisegmental fracture of the distal fibula above the level of the tibiofibular syndesmosis. The arrow points to a widened medial joint space. This is therefore likely to be unstable.

Calcaneal fractures

The calcaneus or heel bone is the largest of the tarsal bones. It supports the total body weight thereby facilitating walking. The subtalar joint (the articulation between the talus and the calcaneus) facilitates inversion and eversion.

Clinical presentation

This is the most commonly injured bone of the hind foot. Fractures are either following a fall from a height or stress fractures in the elderly.

Fractures can be intra-articular (75%) or extra-articular (25%). The most important distinction is whether the subtalar joint is involved, due to its impact on walking.

Imaging

Plain film

These are the initial investigation of choice.

Lateral (Fig. 20.14a)

This view can be carried out for either a specific calcaneal injury or as part of the investigation for an ankle injury. Therefore it is important to always look for a calcaneal fracture when assessing ankle radiographs.

It is important to assess Boehler's angle (normal range 20–40°) on the lateral view as this may be the only indication of an injury.

Axial

This is a specific view of the calcaneus.

CT (Fig. 20.14b)

This is used to provide detailed reconstructions of the full extent of the injury. The surgeons will particularly want to know the extent of damage to the subtalar joint.

MRI

This is only rarely used if there is concern for major soft tissue injuries.

Information for the radiologist

The mechanism as injuries to the hind foot, after a fall from a height, should raise concern for spinal injuries.

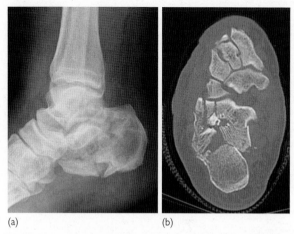

(a)   (b)

Fig. 20.14 A 20-year-old male who jumped from a second floor window and was unable to weight bear after. a) Lateral ankle radiograph showing significant fragmentation of the calcaneus. b) Axial CT image fully demonstrating the true extent of the injury.

Gastrointestinal differential diagnosis

Abdominal calcification

Calcification seen on an abdominal radiograph may be due to calcification of normal structures, or calcification indicating pathology.

Calcification of normal structures

- Ribs (costal cartilage).
- Mesenteric nodes.
- Pelvic veins (phleboliths).
- Prostate.

Abnormal structures to contain calcium

i.e. calcium indicates pathology:

- Pancreas.
- Renal parenchyma.
- Blood vessels and aneurysms.
- Gall bladder (e.g. porcelain gallbladder).
- Uterus (fibroids).

Calcium is pathological

- Biliary calculi.
- Renal calculi.
- Appendicolith.
- Bladder calculi.
- Teratoma.

Ascites

- Cirrhosis.
- Tumours.
- Hypoalbuminaemia.
- Peritonitis.
- Increased pressure in vascular system distal to liver.
- Lymphatic obstruction.

Colonic dilatation

Non-toxic (without abnormal mucosa)

- Mechanical obstruction (e.g. carcinoma).
- Ileus: paralytic/secondary to electrolyte imbalance.
- Pseudo-obstruction: signs or symptoms of LBO but no organic lesion as cause.
- Purgative abuse.

Toxic (with mucosal abnormalities)

- Inflammatory:
  - UC.
  - Crohn's disease.
  - Pseudomembranous colitis.
- Ischaemic colitis.
- Infective (e.g. dysentery).

Pneumoperitoneum

- Perforation of a gas containing viscus:
  - Peptic ulcer.
  - Secondary to inflammation, e.g. diverticulitis, toxic megacolon, necrotizing enterocolitis, appendicitis.
  - Infarction.
  - Malignant neoplasm.
  - Obstruction.
- Iatrogenic. e.g. postoperative, dialysis, etc. (may take a couple of weeks to resorb, but should reduce in amount over time).
- Pneumomediastinum.
- Pneumothorax (pleuroperitoneal fistula).
- Per vaginum.
- Idiopathic.

Pneumatosis intestinalis (gas in the bowel wall)

- Primary (15%):
  - Pneumatosis coli.
- Secondary:
  - Immunosuppressive and steroid therapy.
  - Leukaemia.
  - Colitis and enteritis of any cause (UC, Crohn's, ischaemia, severe infective colitis).
  - Collagen disorders (scleroderma).

Small bowel dilatation

- Mechanical obstruction.
- Paralytic ileus.
- Ischaemia.
- Crohn's disease.
- Radiotherapy.
- Lymphoma.

Strictures

Oesophageal

Strictures of the oesophagus can be separated into smooth and irregular, as they appear at contrast swallow studies.

Smooth
- Inflammatory:
  - Peptic.
  - Scleroderma.
  - Corrosives.
  - Iatrogenic, e.g. after chronic NG tube.
- Neoplastic:
  - Carcinoma (occasionally squamous carcinoma).
  - Mediastinal tumours.
  - Leiomyoma.
- Achalasia.

Irregular
- Neoplastic:
  - Carcinoma.
  - Leiomyosarcoma.
  - Carcinosarcoma.
  - Lymphoma.
- Inflammatory:
  - Reflux (more commonly smooth).
  - Crohn's disease.
- Iatrogenic:
  - Radiotherapy.
  - Fundoplication.

Small bowel
- Adhesions.
- Crohn's disease.
- Ischaemia.
- Radiation.
- Tumours.

Large bowel
- Neoplastic:
  - Carcinoma.
  - Lymphoma.
- Inflammatory:
  - UC, Crohn's, radiotherapy, diverticulosis.
- Ischaemia:
  - Commonest site is splenic flexure at the vascular watershed area.
- Infective:
  - e.g. TB.
- Extrinsic masses:
  - Inflammatory, tumours, endometriosis.

Gastrointestinal presenting syndromes

Upper abdominal pain

Differential diagnosis

- Gastritis.
- Stomach/duodenal ulceration.
- Cholecystitis/cholangitis.
- Pancreatitis.
- Subphrenic abscess.
- Viscus perforation.
- Stomach cancer.
- Liver cancer.
- Pancreatic cancer.

Imaging

The differential diagnosis of upper abdominal pain is wide and the choice of appropriate investigation is guided by obtaining a good clinical history and examination to identify typical features associated with certain conditions.

Investigations utilized in upper abdominal pain include plain radiography, abdominal ultrasound, OGD, and CT. OGD is not an imaging modality and is best suited to investigation of possible gastritis and peptic ulcer disease.

Plain radiographs (erect chest radiograph and abdominal radiograph) may be helpful as the initial investigation to assess for intestinal obstruction or viscus perforation. They can also provide additional information on the presence of gallstones or renal calculi.

TA ultrasonography is the investigation of choice in hepatobiliary or gallstone disease. It also provides information on other important structures within the abdomen which are interrogated during the scan such as the kidneys, spleen, and aorta. .

CT is being used increasingly for definitive assessment of the abdomen either as a primary modality, usually when the patient is acutely unwell or as a problem-solving tool when initial investigations have either identified an abnormality which requires further evaluation or when the patient's ailment remains unexplained. Owing to its optimal depiction of the solid intra-abdominal viscera, small and large bowel, and vascular tree its main roles are in diagnosing acute pathology in addition to staging and follow-up of chronic illness and malignancy.

Vomiting

Vomiting is a common and non-specific symptom. A myriad of causes can trigger the vomiting centre in the brain, many of which will not require imaging. A careful history of the duration and type of symptoms along with the patient's age and associated symptoms will guide the differential and inform whether imaging is required.

Causes

- GI: gastroenteritis, gastric outlet obstruction, bowel obstruction, ileus, gastroparesis.
- Inflammatory: e.g. appendicitis, acute cholecystitis, pancreatitis.
- CNS: head injury, raised intracranial pressure, meningitis, labyrinthine neuronitis, migraine.
- Metabolic/endocrine: hypercalcaemia, uraemia, hyponatraemia, diabetic ketoacidosis.
- Drugs: chemotherapy, antibiotics, opiates, digoxin.
- Alcohol.
- Other: pregnancy, MI, UTI, psychogenic.

Clinical presentation

History

- Distinguish true vomiting from regurgitation.
- Duration of symptoms: acute, chronic, or recurrent.
- Timing: relation to meals, early morning (pregnancy, raised intracranial pressure).
- Content of vomitus: bile, blood, coffee grounds, faeces.
- Abdominal pain, fever, diarrhoea.
- Constipation.
- Headache, neck stiffness, focal neurology, vertigo.
- Pregnancy symptoms, e.g. amenorrhea.
- Weight loss.
- Previous abdominal surgery: consider obstruction secondary to adhesions.
- Primary malignancy: obstruction or cerebral metastases.

Clinical examination

The most relevant findings to inform imaging are signs of obstruction (high pitched bowel sounds, peritonism or abdominal mass and signs of raised intracranial pressure or focal neurology to indicate a CT head.

Imaging

The type of imaging will be guided by the differential diagnosis and the patient's age. Imaging is not indicated in many causes of vomiting, e.g. gastroenteritis or pregnancy. The main role of imaging is to diagnose or exclude mechanical obstruction or intracranial pathology. Imaging may also play a role in diagnosing inflammatory conditions such as appendicitis.

Plain film

An abdominal radiograph is the first-line investigation in suspected bowel obstruction. Features include dilated bowel proximal to an obstruction with a paucity of gas distally. Look for free gas in associated perforation.

Ultrasound

May be first-line investigation of neonates or infants with vomiting, e.g. ?pyloric stenosis or adults with features of inflammatory causes, e.g. pancreatitis or cholecystitis.

CT

CT head is the investigation of choice in suspected neurogenic vomiting, e.g. post-head injury or in a patient with features of raised intracranial pressure or a known primary malignancy at risk of cerebral metastases.

CT of the abdomen and pelvis is carried out in bowel obstruction to look for the site and cause of obstruction. Other inflammatory causes of vomiting such as appendicitis, pancreatitis, and cholecystitis may be detected.

Fluoroscopy

Upper GI contrast studies are used in suspected gastric outlet obstruction and in children.

Nuclear medicine

Radionuclide gastric emptying study may be used in investigation of unexplained nausea and vomiting.

Jaundice

Jaundice is clinically detectable when the serum bilirubin concentration is in excess of 50µmol/L (with a normal value of <1750µmol/L). It can be due to 'pre-hepatic' causes (haemolysis of red blood cells), 'hepatic' causes (including congenital syndromes, hepatitis, and cirrhosis), and 'post-hepatic' or obstructive causes (obstruction of bile secretion distal to the bile canaliculi by stones, strictures, or carcinoma). Imaging is most useful in this latter group.

Clinical presentation

Patients may present as they notice yellow discoloration of the skin and eyes, with severe itching or with weight loss, dark urine, and steatorrhoea. Abdominal pain may be a feature, mostly in association with the more benign causes of jaundice, although not always. Alternatively, deranged liver function tests may be detected during investigation of other conditions or during routine follow-up or preoperative investigation.

Imaging

Plain films

Gallstones may be visualized in the right upper quadrant. Only 10% of gallstones calcify and are radio-opaque so their absence does not exclude gallbladder pathology. Also, gallstones are a common finding within the population, such that their presence is not necessarily causative. Remember, there could be other findings on the plain films which may point to the cause of jaundice such as metastatic deposits, lung mass, etc.

Ultrasound

The main investigation in jaundiced patients. This allows assessment of liver architecture in cirrhosis, the presence of focal lesions and assessment of the biliary tree (gallstones or bile duct obstruction with duct dilatation). In the case of duct dilatation, ultrasound may suggest a mass in the head of pancreas or duodenum, or filling defects within the biliary system, which will need further imaging with CT or MR cholangiopancreatography (MRCP) depending on the clinical picture. Ultrasound is also used for imaged-guided liver biopsy, and may also detect additional pathology such as ascites, splenomegaly, and allow assessment of the portal vein in chronic liver disease. In infants, choledochal cysts may cause obstructive jaundice or ultrasound may demonstrate a small/absent gallbladder and triangular cord sign in biliary atresia.

CT

Used when obstructive jaundice is present and the likely cause is a malignant process. A staging chest abdomen and pelvis CT should be performed.

Nuclear medicine

In infants with jaundice, a HIDA (hydroxy iminodiacetic acid) scan is used to demonstrate whether any biliary excretion of isotope occurs (it doesn't in the case of biliary atresia).

MRI

MRCP should be performed when ultrasound has shown obstructive jaundice and further delineation of the point of obstruction is needed. Most useful for stone disease, although enough detail is usually present to comment on the pancreas in malignancy. This investigation allows ERCP to be reserved solely for patients who require intervention.

Fluoroscopy

ERCP can be used to perform spincterotomy and stone removal in the case of obstructive jaundice following appropriate imaging. Fluoroscopic transjugular liver biopsy may be necessary if the patient's clotting cannot be corrected enough to allow safe percutaneous biopsy.

Information for the radiologist

- Is the jaundice painful or painless? If painless and the gallbladder is palpable then malignant process is more likely than stone disease (Courvosier's law).
- Do the liver function tests indicate an obstructive or hepatitic picture?
- Are there any other features in the history to suggest stone disease versus malignant process?
- Are there any clues on the plain films to guide further investigation?

Melaena

Melaena is the black tarry faeces that are passed following GI haemorrhage. The black colour occurs as the iron in haemoglobin oxidizes as it passes through the GI tract. Mostly, melaena occurs around 14 hours after bleeding has occurred as it takes around this time for oxidization of the iron to occur, and is usually due to upper GI bleeding such as from the stomach, duodenum, or small bowel (proximal to the ligament of Trietz).

Clinical presentation

Patients may present with symptoms and signs of anaemia and have a positive faecal occult blood test. Following large bleeds, patients may present with signs of shock. The differential diagnosis of melaena is wide, encompassing ulcer disease, variceal bleeding, neoplasm, and vascular lesions. Over the last few years the role of imaging has changed from being purely diagnostic to identifying the site of bleeding and underlying pathology, to playing a key role in treatment of the bleed itself.

Imaging

Endoscopy remains the first-line investigation for patients with acute upper GI bleeds.

CT

However, following a negative endoscopic study, in the presence of active bleeding, a CTA would be appropriate.

Essential diagnostic tool: a rapid, non-invasive, sensitive investigation which allows precise localization of bleeding point with concurrent identification of underlying cause and allows accurate intervention planning. Requires a bleeding rate of around 0.3ml/min. Imaging will show extravasation of high attenuation contrast material into the bowel lumen.

Nuclear medicine

Technetium-labelled red blood cell or sulphur colloid scans can be performed to identify and localize chronic GI bleeding. It is a sensitive test in situations of intermittent bleeding or ongoing low volume blood loss (as low as 0.04ml/min), however, in the acute situation of an active, large GI bleed then endoscopy or CT angiograms are clinically more appropriate.

Angiography

Mostly used for therapeutic embolization of bleeding vessels, although can be diagnostic should other modalities fail to identify any bleeding sites, or the patient is acutely unstable. Bleeding rates as low as 0.5ml/min can be detected. The majority of upper GI bleeds will involve vessels arising from the coeliac axis or superior mesenteric artery. The rich collateral supply from these branches allows safe embolization of a bleeding vessel branch with low risk of ischaemic injury.

Information for the radiologist

- Has the patient had a recent CT or barium study? Retained contrast within the bowel can lead to false positives in CTA.
- How haemodynamically stable is the patient?

Iron deficiency anaemia

Iron deficiency anaemia in the setting of GI disorders is caused by chronic low volume blood loss.

Causes
- GI malignancy.
- Inflammatory: Crohn's and UC.
- Malabsorption syndromes: coeliac disease, Whipple's disease.
- Haematological conditions such as leukaemia and lymphoma.
- Infective: parasitic infections.

Imaging
Plain film
Usually the first modality used to assess the abdomen to identify bowel dilatation or hepatosplenomegaly.

Barium examinations
- These are often performed in the setting of iron deficiency anaemia to assess the GI tract for malignancy, signs of inflammatory bowel disease, or malabsorption.
- Upper GI examinations look at the oesophagus and the stomach.
- Areas of stricturing, bowel wall thickening, mucosal ulceration, and fistulation can be identified with accuracy.

CT
- CT is another common modality to assess the abdomen for iron deficiency anaemia.
- CT has a high sensitivity and specificity for identifying the site of bowel abnormality, any perforation or collections, and is used to stage bowel malignancy.
- CT colonoscopy is a method of imaging the large bowel in a way similar to colonoscopy.
- Origin of masses can be accurately identified and staged.

Information for the radiologist
- Clinical presentation and previous chronic diseases such as Crohn's disease or surgical history.
- Clinical findings.
- Haematological findings, inflammatory markers, tumour markers, and renal function.
- Colonoscopy findings if any.

Diarrhoea

Diarrhoea has many causes. The majority of cases of diarrhoea are infective and do not need imaging.

Causes

- Infective, e.g. *Clostridium difficile*.
- Inflammatory: Crohn's disease and UC.
- Ischaemic colitis.
- Malignancy: carcinoid, colonic carcinoma.

Imaging

Plain film

Often the first modality used to assess the abdomen and will identify bowel dilatation or a large soft tissue mass. Small bowel is identified by the presence of the valvulae conniventes, the folds that traverse the lumen. Large bowel shows interdigitating haustral folds. A search for free air needs to be performed. Finally, if there is concern about inflammatory bowel disease, colonic dilatation, particularly transverse colon, needs to be measured. Thickening of the bowel wall gives an appearance known as 'thumb-printing'.

Small bowel follow through and barium enemas

- May be performed in the setting of chronic diarrhoea to look for small bowel or colonic pathology.
- Areas of stricturing in the small or large bowel, wall thickening, mucosal ulceration, and fistulation can be identified with accuracy.

CT

- CT is another common modality to assess the abdomen in the setting of diarrhoea.
- CT has a high sensitivity and specificity for identifying the site of bowel abnormality, any perforation or collections, and is used to stage bowel malignancy.

MRI

MR enterography is increasingly being used to monitor inflammatory bowel disease to identify abnormal bowel, assess disease activity, and identify complications.

Information for the radiologist

- Clinical presentation and previous chronic diseases such as Crohn's disease or surgical history.
- Clinical findings.
- Inflammatory markers and renal function.
- Colonoscopy findings if any.

Abdominal distension

Abdominal distension may be caused by masses, ascites, or bowel obstruction.

Clinical presentation

- Non-specific abdominal pain.
- Malaise and weight loss.
- Abdominal distension:
  - Soft with signs of obstruction?
  - Mass on palpation.
  - Shifting dullness suggestive of ascites.

Imaging

Plain film

Often the first modality used to assess the abdomen. It will identify bowel dilatation or a large soft tissue mass. If the plain film shows bowel dilatation and clinically the patient is obstructed, CT is the next imaging modality. If there is a suspicion of a mass, either an ultrasound or a CT can be performed.

Ultrasound

- An abdominal ultrasound is performed after fasting for 6 hours, with a full bladder.
- Ultrasound is useful to look at the solid abdominal organs, especially the liver and spleen. The aorta can also be assessed for aneurysms.
- It can also identify any free fluid or ascites.
- Mesenteric and para-aortic lymphadenopathy can often be visualized.
- A TA pelvic scan may show the uterus and ovaries if the bladder is full, alternatively a TV scan may be performed.

CT

CT has a high sensitivity and specificity for identifying the site of bowel obstruction. Masses can be accurately identified and staged.

MRI

MRI is mainly used in assessment of gynaecological masses.

Information for the radiologist

Salient features from the clinical history and examination to point towards a diagnosis.

Weight loss

Weight loss that is unintentional is medically significant. Although a very non-specific symptom, there may be serious underlying pathology. There are a multitude of causative factors ranging from inadequate food intake (loss of appetite, vomiting, dysphagia), to malabsorption (inflammatory bowel disease, chronic pancreatitis, fistulae) and increased metabolism (tumours, chronic infection, endocrine abnormalities).

Clinical presentation

Patients may present having noticed a change in their body habitus or noticed that their clothes are loose. Alternatively, others may have commented on a change in appearance. They may have accompanying symptoms of fatigue, lethargy, GI changes, or features of the underlying disease.

Imaging

Plain film

A CXR is a good initial investigation of weight loss, and may demonstrate primary tumour, metastatic bone disease, cardiac failure, or chronic infection such as TB.

Ultrasound

Diagnostic yield is lower with ultrasound than CT but will show metastatic deposits in the liver if present.

CT

Used to search for occult malignancy, although the sensitivity is often low. Should identify malignant causes such as lymphoma, lung, and GI tumours. May suggest inflammatory bowel disease if the bowel wall is thickened. Chronic chest infection can also be clarified with CT.

Fluoroscopy

A barium swallow can be used to diagnose swallowing problems and upper GI contrast studies are useful in the case of achalasia and oesophageal disease.

Information for the radiologist

Are there any specific symptoms present which may guide investigation?

Gastrointestinal conditions

Oesophageal cancer

- Incidence: 9th commonest cancer (UK). Risk factors: male:female ~5:1, diet, excess alcohol, smoking, achalasia, Plummer–Vinson syndrome, obesity, reflux ± Barrett's oesophagus. 5-year survival poor but improved, around 8%.
- Site: 20% upper, 50% middle, 30% lower oesophagus.
- Pathology: squamous (upper/mid) or adenocarcinoma (lower, incidence rising).

Clinical presentation

Progressive dysphagia, weight loss, chest pain.

TNM staging

- Tis: carcinoma *in situ*.
- T1: invading lamina propria/submucosa.
- T2: invading muscularis propria.
- T3: invading adventitia.
- T4: invasion of adjacent structures.
- Nx: nodes cannot be assessed.
- N0: no node spread.
- N1: regional node metastasis.
- M0: no distant spread.
- M1: distant metastasis.

Imaging

OGD is the investigation of choice, allowing direct visualization, assessment of severity of stenosis and biopsy. Therapeutic in the removal of small tumours/stenting.

Plain film

Generally not helpful, may see widened mediastinum/dilated oesophagus, complications such as aspiration pneumonia, pulmonary metastases.

CT (Fig. 23.1)

CT used for tumour staging, to define the local extent of the tumour, detecting mediastinal invasion, lymphadenopathy, and distant metastases.

Fluoroscopy

Contrast swallow appearances include a mass or an infiltrating lesion causing stenosis, occasionally ulceration and mucosal irregularity.

EUS

EUS is the investigation of choice for local staging. The layers of the oesophageal wall and perioesophageal tissues are visible and therefore depth of tumour invasion and local nodal disease can be determined. Problems arise, however, if a significant oesophageal stenosis exists.

PET

Superior to CT in the detection of loco-regional/distant lymphadenopathy and metastases. Now an important part of preoperative imaging.

Information for the radiologist

Clinical history and duration of symptoms with emphasis of features suggestive of malignancy are essential. Endoscopic level and biopsy results.

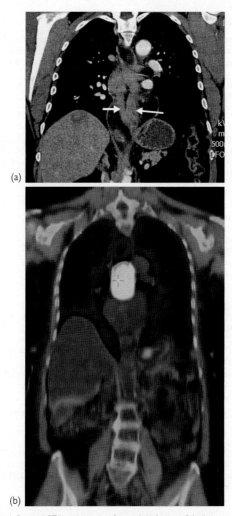

Fig. 23.1 a) Coronal CT showing circumferential thickening of the lower oesophagus (arrowed) in a patient with oesophageal cancer. Note also low attenuation metastasis within the upper liver. b) Coronal image from PET-CT scan, showing intense uptake of an oesophageal tumour (cross). Other areas of increased uptake correspond to physiological uptake.

Gastric cancer

- Incidence: UK 23/100,000/year. Incidence increased at gastro-oesophageal junction, decreased distal and body gastric cancers. Male:female ~2–3:1.
- Adenocarcinoma accounts for >95% malignant tumours stomach, other tumours include lymphoma and GIST.
- Risk factors: *Helicobacter pylori*, atrophic gastritis, smoking, pernicious anaemia, blood group A, adenomatous polyps, diet.
- 5-year survival rates remain low at about 15%.

Clinical presentation

Often non-specific and late. New-onset dyspepsia, dysphagia, vomiting, anorexia, weight loss, or haematemesis warrant investigation. Patients with advanced disease often have constitutional symptoms of anorexia and weight loss.

TNM staging

- Tis: carcinoma *in situ*.
- T1: invading lamina propria/submucosa.
- T2: invading muscularis propria/subserosa.
- T3: penetrates subserosa.
- T4: invasion of adjacent structures.
- N1: metastasis to 1–6 regional nodes.
- N2: metastasis to 7–15 regional nodes.
- N3: metastasis to >15 regional nodes.
- M0: no distant spread.
- M1: distant metastasis.

Imaging

OGD (and biopsy) is the investigation of choice for diagnosing gastric cancer. The role of imaging is in the accurate preoperative staging of the disease once a diagnosis has been established.

Laparoscopy performed in patients considered for radical surgery, as may identify occult peritoneal metastasis.

CT (Fig. 23.2)

CT provides staging information on the tumour mass, loco-regional/distant lymphadenopathy, and metastatic spread of disease.

EUS

In patients with no evidence of distant disease, EUS may be used to evaluate local extent of the tumour as it able to define the individual layers of the gastric wall and thus accurately assess the depth of invasion of the gastric tumour and local invasion.

PET

Role is still being evaluated; may have a role in recurrent disease and assessment of treatment response.

Information for the radiologist

Clinical history and duration of symptoms with emphasis on features consistent with malignancy are essential. Endoscopic evaluation and histological diagnosis is important before embarking upon staging investigations if the patient is a candidate for active treatment.

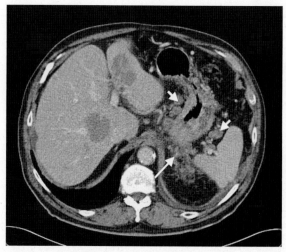

Fig. 23.2 Axial CT showing abnormal thickening of the stomach, with local lymphadenopathy (short arrows), and extension into the perigastric fat (long arrow). Low attenuation lesions within the liver are metastases.

Colonic cancer

- UK: 3rd commonest malignancy; 2nd commonest cancer death. Risk factors: chronic inflammatory bowel disease, hereditary polyposis and non-polyposis syndromes, previous bowel cancer, smoking.
- Majority adenocarcinomas arise in pre-existing adenomatous polyps.

Clinical presentation

- Most tumours arise in the left colon, causing rectal bleeding, altered bowel habit, and colicky pain.
- Right-sided tumours present with iron deficiency anaemia/RIF mass.

TNM staging

- Tis: carcinoma *in situ*.
- T1: invading submucosa.
- T2: invading muscularis propria.
- T3: invading through muscularis propria.
- T4: invasion of adjacent structures/perforates peritoneum.
- N0: no node spread.
- N1: metastasis in 1–3 regional nodes.
- N2: metastasis in ≥ 4 regional lymph nodes.
- M0: no distant spread.
- M1: distant metastasis.

Imaging

Colonoscopy is the first-line test for tumour detection and biopsy. Imaging studies are less invasive, indicated in patients unable to undergo/failed colonoscopy. CT colonography (CTC) has overtaken double contrast barium enema (DCBE) as the colorectal imaging method of choice, with better sensitivity, and specificity approaching colonoscopy.

Plain film

Useful in suspected acute bowel obstruction (presenting feature in <20% of tumours), perforation, and detection of pulmonary metastases.

CT (Fig. 23.3)

CTC requires bowel preparation and gaseous distension to allow visibility of intraluminal lesions. It may show extramural infiltration or synchronous lesions. Extra-colonic structures can also be evaluated. Staging is by CT chest, abdomen, and pelvis to assess local stage and metastases.

Fluoroscopy

DCBE may demonstrate a malignant polyp as an intraluminal filling defect, advanced tumours have annular appearance ('apple-core' deformity). If acutely obstructed, stenting may have a role.

Nuclear medicine

Combined PET/CT is a useful adjunct in detection of recurrent cancer. Isotope bone scan can be performed for suspected bone metastases.

Information for the radiologist

- If there are symptoms of acute obstruction.
- If known tumour, exact location, or suspicion from clinical signs, e.g. anaemia.
- CEA.
- Relevant risk factors.

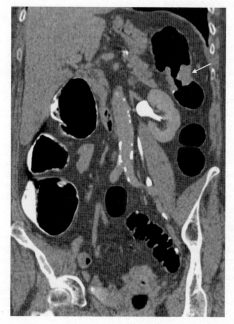

Fig. 23.3 Coronal CT showing large bowel obstruction secondary to proximal descending colonic tumour. Endoluminal view from the CT colonoscopy showing tumour.

Rectal cancer

- Approximately 20% of colorectal cancers occur in the rectum; majority are adenocarcinomas.
- Although risk factors are similar to colonic tumours, investigation and treatment are different.

Clinical presentation

Change in bowel habit (diarrhoea or constipation), tenesmus, bleeding, non-specific symptoms, e.g. tiredness, weight loss.

Imaging

Plain film

Useful in suspected acute bowel obstruction, perforation, and detection of pulmonary metastases.

Ultrasound

Transrectal ultrasound is better at depicting the layers of the rectal wall than MRI, useful in the assessment of early wall involvement and selecting T1 N0 tumours for local excision.

CT

May be useful if the rectal lesion cannot be traversed with the colonoscope, to evaluate the rest of the bowel, as synchronous carcinomas are seen in 5% of cases, and synchronous adenomas in 27–55% cases. Extra-colonic structures can also be evaluated. Staging is by CT chest, abdomen, and pelvis to assess local stage and metastases.

MRI (Fig. 23.4)

Indicated for staging rectal tumours, performed to assess involvement of mesorectal fascia and suitability for total mesorectal excision. Nodal/venous involvement is also assessed and the need for neoadjuvant treatment.

Fluoroscopy

DCBE may demonstrate a malignant polyp as an intraluminal filling defect, advanced tumours have annular appearance ('apple-core' deformity). If acutely obstructed, stenting may have a role for more proximal rectal tumours.

Nuclear medicine

Combined PET/CT is a useful adjunct in detection of recurrent rectal cancer.

Information for the radiologist

- Level of tumour from the anal verge.
- Any contraindication to MRI.
- CEA level.

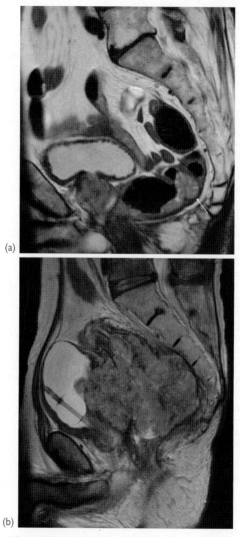

Fig. 23.4 a) Sagittal MRI scan of a patient with an early villous tumour of the posterior wall of the lower rectum (arrow). b) Sagittal MRI showing locally advanced tumour of the rectum, extending anteriorly into the bladder and posteriorly to the sacrum.

Gastrointestinal lymphoma

- Site: stomach >small bowel >colon >pancreas >oesophagus.
- Usually diffuse large B-cell (~50%)/marginal zone/MALT (~40%).
- Risk factors: coeliac disease, immunoproliferative small-intestinal disease (alpha-chain disease), chronic lymphatic lymphoma, previous extra-intestinal lymphoma.

Clinical presentation

- General malaise and anorexia.
- Symptoms of intestinal obstruction if the affected bowel lumen is compromised.
- May give rise to intussusception.
- Dysphagia if the oesophagus is affected.

Imaging

For diagnosis, monitoring of response or complications of therapy.

Plain film

Chest radiograph may demonstrate lymphadenopathy.

Fluoroscopy

Barium swallow/meal/enema may show large irregular mural filling defects/ fine submucosal nodules/thickening of folds.

Ultrasound

- Can assess spleen/liver, but difficult to assess infiltrative disease.
- Good for assessment of superficial nodal masses, and ultrasound-guided biopsies can be performed to gain tissue diagnosis.

CT (Fig. 23.5)

Most useful investigation. The extent of spread of the mass and evaluation of sites of neoplastic involvement can be demonstrated.

PET

May be used to identify active disease prior to, or post treatment.

Information for the radiologist

- Clinical symptoms if primary presentation—therefore choice of most appropriate radiological investigation can be made.
- Biopsy results.
- Relevant past medical history, e.g. coeliac disease.

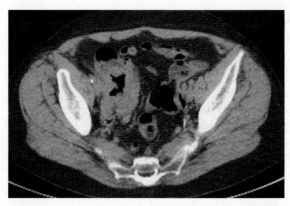

Fig. 23.5 Axial CT showing circumferential thickening of the caecum, in a patient with lymphoma. The bowel is thickened, with a dilated lumen, and there is no proximal obstruction.

Liver tumours

- *Benign:* haemangiomas are the commonest liver lesions, along with hepatic adenomas and focal nodular hyperplasia.
- *Malignant:* hepatocellular cancer (HCC) is one of the world's commonest cancers. It is associated with chronic liver disease, particularly hepatitis B and C.

Metastases can occur in the liver commonly from colon, lung, breast, pancreas and stomach cancers.

Clinical presentation

- Pain (as the liver capsule is stretched).
- Deranged LFTs or jaundice.
- Anorexia or weight loss.
- Many liver tumours are small and clinically undetected. In metastatic disease, symptoms may only be apparent from the primary tumour.

Imaging

Ultrasound

Good first-line test, used for follow-up of patients at risk of HCC. Used for image guided-biopsy.

CT (Fig. 23.6)

- Follow-up of patients with a known primary malignancy that is known to have spread to the liver.
- Different timing of contrast enhancement may be used depending on the type of tumour.

MRI

Excellent tool for problem-solving of liver tumours if a lesion identified on ultrasound or CT requires further characterization.

Information for the radiologist

- Relevant medical history, e.g. malignancy, cirrhosis, long-term use of the oral contraceptive pill (adenoma risk factor).
- Haematology and biochemistry results: especially LFTs, and clotting if a biopsy is to be performed.

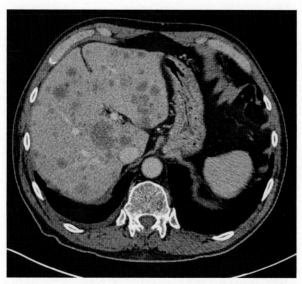

Fig. 23.6 Axial CT showing multiple low attenuation lesions within the liver, in keeping with metastases.

Cholangiocarcinoma

- >95% adenocarcinoma, arise from biliary epithelium.
- Risk factors: age (>60 years), chronic inflammation, e.g. primary sclerosing cholangitis, viral hepatitis, cirrhosis and liver fluke (parasitic) infestation only account for a few.
- Classified as intrahepatic, hilar (Klatskin) or extrahepatic (most common).

Clinical presentation

- Often progress insidiously and present late.
- Poor prognosis: 5-year survival rate <5%.
- Extrahepatic present with painless obstructive jaundice.
- Intrahepatic tumours present with non-specific symptoms such as anorexia, weight loss, abdominal pain.
- Cholangitis is an unusual presentation.

TNM staging

- TIS: carcinoma *in situ*.
- T1a: invades mucosa.
- T1b: invades muscularis.
- T2: invades perimuscular connective tissue.
- T3: invades adjacent structures.
- N0: no node spread.
- N1: metastasis in cystic duct/peridochal/hilar nodes.
- N2: metastasis in peripancreatic, periduodenal, periportal, coeliac, or superior mesenteric nodes.
- M0: no distant spread.
- M1: distant metastasis (including lymph node metastases beyond N2).

Imaging

Ultrasound (Fig. 23.7a)

First-line investigation for obstructive jaundice. The tumour is rarely seen, its location correlates with point of biliary tree calibre change. Detection of metastases, biliary duct dilatation, and exclusion of gallstones.

CT (Fig. 23.7b)

Used in staging of cholangiocarcinomas, to identify the cause of biliary obstruction, lymph nodes, and metastases.

MRI

Superior to CT in identifying intraductal lesions and their extent owing to its greater soft tissue contrast resolution.

ERCP

- ERCP may establish the diagnosis by obtain brushings, and intraductal biopsies. Therapeutic procedures, such as stent insertion to relieve biliary obstruction may be performed.
- EUS is sensitive for assessing loco-regional lymphadenopathy and biopsy.

PET

PET remains an emerging technique for staging cholangiocarcinoma.

Information for the radiologist

Duration of symptoms with emphasis on features suggestive of malignancy. Severity of obstructive jaundice is useful (degree of derangement LFTs). Signs suggestive of cholangitis (raised WCC, CRP) should prompt urgent discussion with a view to ERCP.

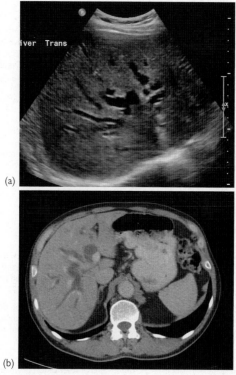

(a)

(b)

Fig. 23.7 a) Ultrasound image showing dilated intrahepatic ducts. b) Axial CT showing dilated intrahepatic ducts, secondary to a filling defect within the duct, washings at ERCP confirmed cholangiocarcinoma.

Pancreatic cancer

- Incidence: 11th commonest cancer in UK and rising.
- Risk factors include smoking, age, chronic pancreatitis, diabetes mellitus, obesity.
- 90% are adenocarcinomas arising from pancreatic duct epithelium. 5-year survival <2%.

Clinical presentation

Often present with advanced disease. 80% of pancreatic tumours arise in the pancreatic head; classically present with painless obstructive jaundice (Courvoisier's law—if palpable gallbladder jaundice is unlikely due to gallstones). Constitutional symptoms are common. Late onset diabetes and pancreatitis are recognized but infrequent presentations.

TNM staging

- T1: tumour limited to pancreas ≤2cm.
- T2: tumour limited to pancreas >2cm.
- T3: tumour extends beyond the pancreas without involvement of the coeliac axis or superior mesenteric artery.
- T4: tumour involvement of the coeliac axis or superior mesenteric artery.
- N0: no regional lymph node metastasis.
- N1: regional lymph node metastasis.
- M0: no distant spread.
- M1: distant metastasis.

Imaging

Ultrasound

Primary investigation in obstructive jaundice. The liver, biliary tree, and gallbladder are assessed for metastases, biliary duct dilatation, and for the exclusion of gallstones respectively. Views of the pancreas often limited.

CT (Fig. 23.8)

Triple-phase CT of the pancreas is the modality of choice for detecting and staging pancreatic cancer. Useful in assessment of resectability (local invasion of major vascular structures). Accurately identifies loco-regional/distant lymphadenopathy and metastatic disease.

MRI

MRI similar performance as CT, better at characterization of small lesions and assessing resectability.

EUS

Benefit of enabling biopsy along with tumour staging.

ERCP

For stent insertion, brushings and cytology.

PET

Useful for lesion detection when CT not identified mass, and detection of occult metastases.

Information for the radiologist

Clinical history and duration of symptoms are important with emphasis on features suggestive of malignancy. An indicator of the severity of obstructive jaundice is useful. Symptoms/signs and biochemical parameters (raised WCC, CRP) suggestive of cholangitis should prompt urgent discussion with a view to ERCP.

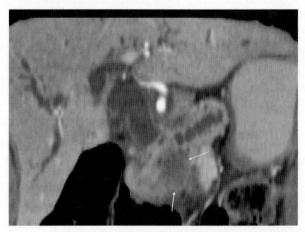

Fig. 23.8 Coronal CT image from a patient with pancreatic cancer. The CT shows 'double duct' dilatation, i.e. dilatation of the intra- and extrahepatic biliary tree, and pancreatic duct, secondary to a large low attenuation mass within the pancreas (arrowed).

Achalasia, hiatus hernia, and reflux

- Achalasia: oesophageal motility disorder with failure of relaxation of the lower oesophageal sphincter and disordered peristalsis.
- Hiatus hernia: protrusion of stomach into the thoracic cavity. Two types; sliding (commonest) and rolling.
- Gastro-oesophageal reflux disease (GORD): range of symptoms caused by reflux of gastric acid into the lower oesophagus. Often secondary to lower oesophageal sphincter incompetence.

Clinical presentation

Difficult to discriminate reliably between these diagnoses owing to cross-over in symptomatology. Heartburn, acid reflux often worse after meals and on lying flat, dysphagia and chest pain are common. Dysphagia to solids/liquids with regurgitation of food is suggestive of achalasia.

Imaging

Several imaging techniques available to aid diagnosis including endoscopy, barium studies, and radionuclide techniques. Oesophageal manometry and pH measurements are physiological investigations, the latter of which is the gold standard for diagnosing oesophageal motility disorders but is limited by invasiveness, time-consumption, and lack of availability.

Plain film

Often incidental finding. Retrocardiac soft tissue density ± air-fluid levels are suggestive of a hiatus hernia. Dilated oesophagus may be seen in achalasia.

Fluoroscopy (Fig. 23.9)

Double-contrast barium swallow is sensitive for investigation of oesophageal disorders and superior to endoscopy in identifying motility disorders. Accurate at identifying achalasia ('bird's beak' appearance), classifying hernias and visualization of reflux of barium.

Nuclear medicine

Rarely used in assessment of motility disorders and GORD. Ingestion of ^{99m}Tc radiolabelled foods/liquids.

Information for the radiologist

Features suggestive of malignancy, such as progressive dysphagia, anorexia, weight loss, and anaemia is essential.

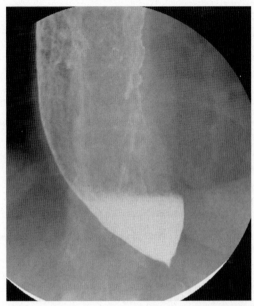

Fig. 23.9 Double-contrast swallow shows abnormal dilatation of the oesophagus, tapering to a 'bird's beak' narrowing at the gastro-oesophageal junction.

Appendicitis

- Common cause of acute abdominal pain.
- May require emergency surgery to prevent complications of perforation and peritonitis.

Clinical presentation

- Highest incidence age 10–19 years.
- Classical presentation (<50%) central abdominal pain migrating to right iliac fossa, accompanied by fever, anorexia, nausea, and vomiting.
- Presentation in the very young and the elderly may be less typical with a rapidly progressing course.
- Clinical signs: rebound tenderness, right iliac fossa tenderness (McBurney's point), Rovsing's sign (right iliac fossa pain on palpation of left iliac fossa).

Imaging

Plain film

- Appendicolith seen in <10% of cases.
- Non-specific features include lumbar scoliosis concave to the right, loss of the right pro-peritoneal fat stripe or psoas shadow, and distal small bowel obstruction.

Ultrasound

- High-frequency linear probe using graded compression.
- Highly operator dependant, most useful in the young/thin.
- Classic findings are of a blind ending, non-compressible tubular structure with diameter >6mm and hyperaemia.
- Additional findings may include localized fluid collection or abscess and an appendicolith.
- Retro-caecal appendix may be difficult to identify.

CT (Fig. 23.10)

Considered by many to be the gold standard investigation but used with caution in children and women of childbearing age due to radiation risks. CT features include a distended, enhancing appendix measuring >6mm in diameter, lack of oral contrast in the appendiceal lumen and stranding of the peri-appendiceal fat.

Information for the radiologist

- Clinical features of pyrexia and raised inflammatory markers.
- In females: last menstrual period and any gynaecological symptoms.

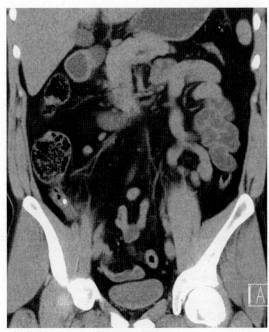

Fig. 23.10 Coronal CT showing thickening of the wall of the appendix, and calcified appendicolith within. Note the peri-appendiceal inflammatory changes.

Cholecystitis/cholangitis

- Gallstones are extremely common, especially in females.
- Acute cholecystitis is inflammation of the gallbladder secondary to gallstone impaction.
- Acute cholangitis is inflammation of the biliary ducts secondary to ascending infection *(Escherichia coli, Klebsiella* spp., *Enterococci)* in the presence of biliary obstruction, and a potentially fatal condition.

Clinical presentation

- Acute cholecystitis: right upper quadrant pain (Murphy's sign) ± right shoulder tip pain. Nausea and vomiting.
- Acute cholangitis: right upper quadrant pain, obstructive jaundice and rigors (Charcot's triad). Nausea and vomiting. Severe systemic upset not infrequent. Grossly deranged LFTs with high bilirubin and raised CRP/ESR.

Imaging

Ultrasound (Fig. 23.11a)

Initial investigation for suspected gallbladder and biliary pathology. Excellent for identification of gallstones and confirmation of cholecystitis and the presence of biliary duct dilatation.

MRI (MRCP)

Non-invasive evaluation of biliary duct dilatation, strictures and intraductal filling defects. Reserved for cases when clinical suspicion is high for gallstone related pathology but initial investigations are equivocal.

Fluoroscopy (ERCP)

Optimal therapeutic option in acute cholangitis. Assessment of biliary tree and identification of cause of obstruction and treatment with sphincterotomy and stent insertion to relieve obstruction.

CT (Fig. 23.11b)

Reserved for atypical cases or when complications are suspected such as emphysematous cholecystitis.

Information for the radiologist

Clinical history, relevant examination findings and supportive biochemical findings (LFTs, raised WCC, CRP/ESR) are essential. Features suggestive of cholangitis warrant urgent discussion with a view to ERCP.

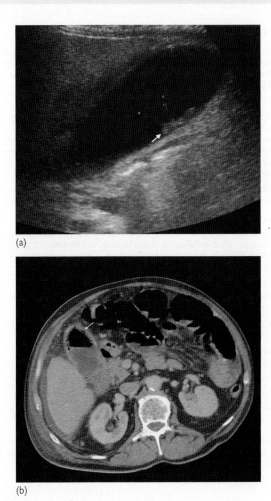

(a)

(b)

Fig. 23.11 a) Ultrasound showing thickened gallbladder wall (asterisk), and dependent stones (arrow), in a patient with marked tenderness (Murphy's sign positive). b) Axial CT of another patient showing thickened gall bladder wall, with gas within (arrow), in keeping with emphysematous cholecystitis. Marked surrounding inflammatory changes of the fat, and ascites around the liver.

Stomach/duodenal ulceration

Ulceration occurring within the acid environment of the stomach or duodenum. Common in elderly. Duodenal ulcers>gastric ulcers. Risk factors: *Helicobacter pylori*, drugs (aspirin, NSAIDs, steroids, bisphosphonate), smoking, stress.

Clinical presentation

Gastric ulcers classically present with intermittent, burning epigastric pain occurring shortly after meals with minimal relief by food or antacids. Duodenal ulceration typically causes pain before meals and at night, relieved by bland foods and alkalis such as milk. However, there is much symptom overlap and often ulcer type differentiation cannot be made on history alone.

ALARM symptoms: anaemia; loss weight; anorexia; recent onset; melaena/haematemesis; swallowing difficulties.

Imaging

OGD is the investigation of choice for diagnosing peptic ulcer disease. In addition to direct visualization, tissue biopsies can be taken to assess for *H. pylori* infection and malignancy. Therapeutic intervention for bleeding ulcers is also commonly performed.

Plain film

Pneumoperitoneum if perforation has occurred.

CT (Fig. 23.12)

Used for identification of complications, such as abscess formation, detection of free gas.

Fluoroscopy

Traditional test for ulceration was a barium study, but this has been superseded by endoscopy, which allows biopsy and direct visualization.

Information for the radiologist

A clear, concise history outlining pertinent risk factors, i.e. relevant medications, concerning features such as anorexia or weight loss and supportive examination findings or biochemical derangement, i.e. microcytic anaemia is ideal. In the acute situation, if a viscus perforation is suspected, clinical history and examination findings, relevant blood tests, i.e. serum lactate and plain radiograph findings are essential.

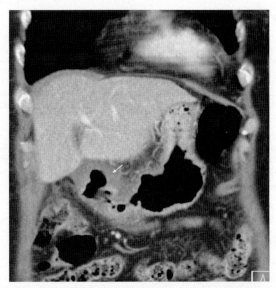

Fig. 23.12 Coronal CT showing thickening of the distal stomach (arrow) with surrounding inflammatory change, in a patient with a locally perforated peptic ulcer.

Crohn's disease

Chronic recurrent inflammatory condition of the GI tract of unknown aetiology, characterized by transmural inflammation. Lesions may occur anywhere in the GI tract but are most common in the small bowel (especially the terminal ileum) and the colon. Discontinuous and asymmetric involvement is characteristic. The earliest pathological feature is apthoid ulceration which progresses to frank ulceration. Complications include fistula formation, abscesses, and strictures. It may also cause complications outside of the GI tract.

Clinical presentation

Peak incidence 15–25 years. A 2nd peak has been reported in the 50–80-year age group. Onset may be insidious. Chronic diarrhoea which may be bloody, abdominal pain and weight loss are common presenting symptoms.

Complications

- Hepatobiliary: hepatic steatosis, gallstones, primary sclerosing cholangitis.
- Pancreatitis.
- Urinary tract: nephrolithiasis, enterovesical fistula.
- Musculoskeletal: arthritis.

Imaging

Imaging was traditionally by contrast studies (DCBE and SBFT), however these have been replaced by non-ionizing investigations magnetic resonance enterography (MRE) and ultrasound.

Ultrasound

Thickened, hyperaemic small bowel loops, most useful in imaging young thin patients.

MRE (Fig. 23.13)

Demonstrates disease distribution, activity, response to treatment, enteric and extra-enteric complications, e.g. perianal fistulae.

CT

Used in acute presentations to detect complications, disease extent and detection of extra-enteric complications.

Information for the radiologist

Due to the nature of the disease, patients with Crohn's disease are likely to undergo repeated examinations in the course of their treatment, and as a result investigations should only be performed when they will help guide management.

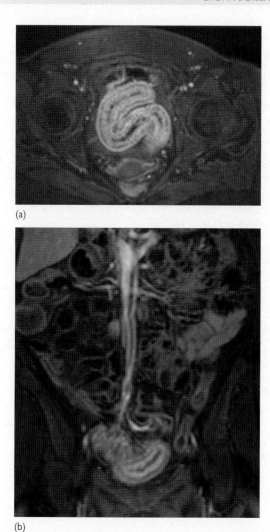

(a)

(b)

Fig. 23.13 a) Axial and b) coronal images from a MRE study. There is a loop of abnormal pelvic small bowel showing wall thickening, mucosal enhancement and engorged vessels in keeping with active disease.

Ulcerative colitis

Relapsing and remitting continuous non-transmural inflammation of the rectum (proctitis ~50%) and colon (left-sided ~30%; pancolitis ~20%), may be associated 'backwash ileitis' (inflammation of the terminal ileum). Histological diagnosis from endoscopic biopsy.

Clinical presentation

- Gradual onset diarrhoea. Abdominal pain is common. Systemic symptoms during attacks.
- Extra-enteric signs seen at imaging: arthritis, sacro-iliitis, ankylosing spondylitis, fatty liver, PSC, cholangiocarcinoma, amyloidosis.
- Complications: perforation, bleeding, toxic megacolon, venous thrombosis, colonic cancer (risk ~15% with pancolitis for 20 years).

Imaging

Imaging used in diagnosis, monitoring therapy response or complications.

Plain film (Fig. 23.14)

Abdominal X-ray: acute setting only, looking for perforation, abnormal dilatation (toxic megacolon >6cm), thickening of bowel wall and thumb-printing (mucosal oedema).

CT

In acute setting may be used to confirm colitis and extent of disease. May help to differentiate causes of colitis. Demonstration of complications.

MRI

Used in some centres as an alternative to CT for imaging the colon. Useful in investigating specific complications, e.g. primary sclerosing cholangitis/cholangiocarcinoma, sacro-iliitis. In pancolitis with an equivocal biopsy MRE can be used to help differentiate UC from Crohn's disease.

Fluoroscopy

DCBE contraindicated in the acute setting due to risk of perforation!

Information for the radiologist

- Clinical symptoms if primary presentation—therefore choice of most appropriate radiological investigation can be made. Information on any biopsy results.
- Relevant past medical history, e.g. coeliac disease.

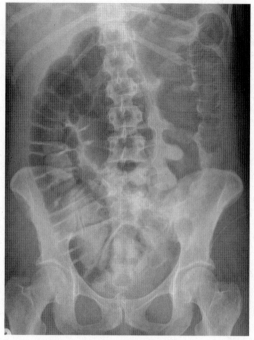

Fig. 23.14 Abdominal radiograph showing grossly thickened wall of the transverse colon, with characteristic 'thumb-printing'.

Infective colitis

Aetiology: bacterial *(Salmonella, Shigella, Campylobacter, E. coli)*, protozoal *(Amoebiasis)* and viral (herpes and *Cytomegalovirus*). Increasing incidence in UK due to rise in foreign travel and use of broad-spectrum antibiotics (pseudomembranous colitis).

Clinical presentation

Diarrhoea, which may be bloody, non-specific abdominal pain, and pyrexia, associated with anorexia, malaise, and dehydration. Hypotension, tachycardia, and impaired renal function are indicators of severity.

Imaging

Stool MC&S is the investigation of choice for diagnosing infective colitis with blood tests used to aid assessment of severity. Sigmoidoscopy/colonoscopy are first-line imaging techniques, as they are more sensitive than radiological investigations for mucosal changes of ulceration and haemorrhage, and to permit biopsy.

Radiology is reserved for assessing the extent and severity of disease and to identify complications.

Plain film

Initial investigation for complications, e.g. colonic dilatation and toxic megacolon (fulminant colitis) or perforation.

CT (Fig. 23.15)

Disease extent can be appreciated on CT which may range from a localized process to a pancolitis. Toxic megacolon and colonic perforation can be accurately identified in addition to further complications such as intra-abdominal collections and liver abscesses.

Ultrasound

Alternative to CT for identification of liver abscesses and performing percutaneous intervention. Identification of bowel wall thickening may be possible.

Information for the radiologist

Stool specimen analysis is paramount. Results of additional investigations such as plain radiographs or colonoscopy. Reasons for further investigation need to be explained. Patients may need to be imaged at the end of the list due to the infection risk.

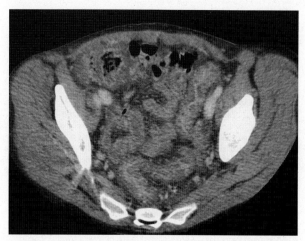

Fig. 23.15 Axial CT showing diffusely thickened colon, in keeping with colitis in a patient with *Clostridium difficile* infection.

Small bowel obstruction

~20% of acute surgical admissions. Subdivided into partial or complete, simple or strangulated. If not diagnosed promptly, vascular compromise can lead to bowel ischaemia, with high mortality. The leading cause in developed countries is postoperative adhesions, other causes include hernia, tumour, inflammatory bowel disease, and volvulus.

Clinical presentation

Four cardinal features are pain, vomiting, distension and constipation. Obstruction of bowel leads to proximal dilatation secondary to accumulation of gastrointestinal secretions and swallowed air. This leads to increased peristalsis both proximal and distal to the obstruction, with initial frequent loose stools and flatus. Increasing small-bowel distension leads to increased intraluminal pressures. Vomiting occurs if obstruction is proximal. Constipation occurs as normal transit of bowel contents is not possible (may be absent early).

Imaging

Plain film
- Abdominal x-ray (Fig. 23.16a): dilated loops of small bowel (>2.5cm) ± air fluid levels, identified by their central position and presence of valvulae conniventes. Gas trapped in the valvulae (string of pearls sign) may also be identified. Depending on degree of obstruction, there may be paucity of gas throughout the colon. Cause/complications of SBO may be identified, e.g. hernia, perforation, or ischaemia.
- Erect CXR: if there is any suspicion of perforation.

CT (Fig. 23.16b)
Confirms the presence, severity and cause of obstruction. Diagnosis is by identifying dilated loops of small bowel and a transition point with collapsed loops of distal bowel, excluding ileus. Complications of obstruction such as ischaemia or perforation can be identified.

Information for the radiologist
- Relevant medical history, e.g. previous operations, hernia.
- Any clinical evidence of developing ischaemia?

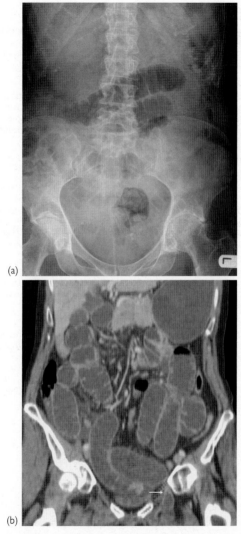

Fig. 23.16 a) Abdominal X-ray showing gas-filled loops of centrally-placed, dilated small bowel. b) Coronal CT showing dilated fluid-filled small bowel loops, secondary to an obstructed left inguinal hernia (arrow).

Large bowel obstruction

Obstruction may be luminal, within the bowel wall or extraluminal. Left-sided obstruction >right.

Common causes include tumour, abscess, diverticular disease, volvulus, and extrinsic compression from pelvic tumour.

Clinical presentation

Features of obstruction: pain, vomiting, distension, and constipation. These features may vary according to the location, age, underlying pathology, or presence of ischaemia. The more distal the obstruction, the longer the interval between onset of symptoms and appearance of nausea and vomiting.

Imaging

Plain film (Fig. 23.17a)

Supine abdominal X-ray: dilated loops of gas-filled large bowel, recognized by their peripheral position and presence of haustral folds. In a minority of patients the ileocaecal valve is competent and in spite of increasing colonic pressure, the small bowel is not distended. When the valve is incompetent, the caecum and ascending colon may not be distended and there may be marked small bowel distension.

CT (Fig. 23.17b)

Confirms the presence of a mechanical obstruction and to look for the underlying cause. In the presence of a tumour it may be used to plan for surgical treatment. Complications of obstruction such as perforation or ischaemia can also be identified.

Fluoroscopy

Water-soluble enema can be performed to confirm the presence of mechanical obstruction/exclude pseudo-obstruction/ileus, although its role is second line to CT.

Information for the radiologist

- Relevant medical history, e.g. oncological disease/previous sigmoid volvulus.
- Whether there is clinical evidence of developing ischaemia.

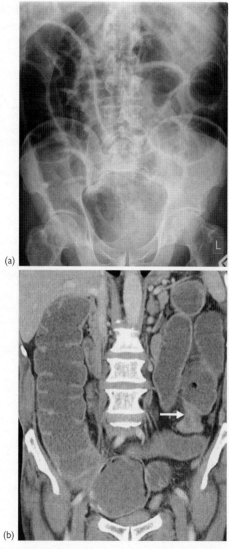

Fig. 23.17 a) Abdominal radiograph showing dilated loops of large and small bowel, secondary to an obstructing distal colonic tumour. b) Coronal CT showing the obstructing tumour (arrow).

Paralytic ileus and pseudo-obstruction

Paralytic ileus occurs when intestinal peristalsis ceases and there is an accumulation of fluid and gas in the bowel, leading to non-specific dilatation of both small and large bowel mimicking obstruction. Causes include postoperative ileus, electrolyte disturbance, and peritonitis. A localized small bowel ileus affecting only 1 or 2 adjacent loops ('sentinel loops') can occur in response to a local inflammatory process, such as acute pancreatitis.

Pseudo-obstruction refers to large bowel distention resulting from chronic impairment of motility. Patients are usually elderly, often on anticholinergics. The degree of colonic distension may be severe enough to cause caecal perforation. Surgical intervention is occasionally necessary.

Clinical presentation

Paralytic ileus and pseudo-obstruction present with abdominal distension, usually without pain (unlike in mechanical obstruction). Patients may or may not continue to pass flatus and stool.

Imaging

Plain film (Fig. 23.18a)

In paralytic ileus, distended small and large bowel loops are seen with the degree of distension varying from local dilatation of a short length of bowel to distension of the entire intestine. When there is generalized bowel distension, the appearances cannot usually be distinguished on plain radiograph alone from low grade large bowel obstruction.

In pseudo-obstruction, the large bowel is dilated all the way to the rectum, and the small bowel may be distended as well. The caecum may exceed the critical diameter of 9cm when perforation is imminent.

CT (Fig. 23.18b)

This is sometimes required to exclude mechanical obstruction and to prevent unnecessary surgery.

Fluoroscopy

Water-soluble enema may be required to exclude mechanical obstruction, but CT is usually the preferred method of investigation.

Information for the radiologist

- Presenting symptoms and signs.
- Any recent surgery.

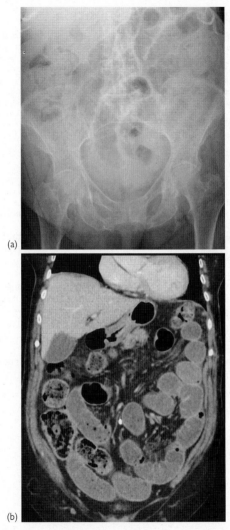

Fig. 23.18 a) Abdominal X-ray showing prominent gas-filled loops of small bowel, with a normal gas pattern in the large bowel, in keeping with ileus. b) Coronal CT from the same patient showing fluid-filled loops of small bowel, with no transition point to collapsed bowel. Normal faeces and gas within the large bowel. This is in keeping with ileus.

Gastrointestinal perforation

Complete penetration of the wall of the oesophagus, stomach, or bowel, resulting in the intestinal contents in the thorax or abdomen, depending on the site of perforation. Potentially a surgical emergency. Intestinal perforation results in bacterial contamination of the abdominal cavity, gastric perforation can lead to a chemical peritonitis.

Causes: iatrogenic (following a procedure, e.g. endoscopy/colonoscopy), spontaneous (duodenal ulcer, appendicitis, diverticulitis, tumour), traumatic.

Clinical presentation

These depend on the site of perforation:
- Chest pain/dysphagia (if oesophageal).
- Severe abdominal pain/rigidity (due to peritonitis).
- Sepsis (depending on organ which has perforated).

Imaging

Plain film
- Erect CXR (Fig. 23.19): pneumoperitoneum or pneumomediastinum, pleural effusion, subcutaneous emphysema of the neck.
- Supine abdominal X-ray: Rigler's sign (gas on both sides of the bowel wall), or outlining of the falciform ligament. In infants, free gas collects centrally producing a rounded translucency (football sign).

CT
More sensitive at identifying free gas and suggesting its origin—large amounts of free gas suggest perforation of large bowel, large amounts of fluid indicate a small bowel perforation. May see oral contrast extravasation.

Fluoroscopy
Used less now as increased use of CT. Water soluble contrast studies:
- Swallow (for suspected oesophageal perforation).
- Enema (for lower GI perforation/to check anastomotic sites post lower GI surgery).

Information for the radiologist
- History of recent procedures, e.g. endoscopy.
- Whether patient is able to take oral preparation (for CT).

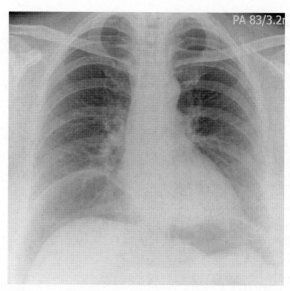

Fig. 23.19 Erect CXR showing free gas under the diaphragm in a patient with perforated duodenal ulcer.

Subphrenic abscess

Majority occur following surgery, and high mortality associated with these abscesses can be reduced by their early diagnosis and management. The subphrenic space extends from the diaphragm above to the transverse mesocolon below and can be divided into 2:

- Left subphrenic space: the commonest cause is following operation on the stomach, the tail of pancreas, the spleen, or splenic flexure of the colon.
- Right subphrenic space: common causes are perforating cholecystitis, perforated duodenal ulcer, and appendicitis.

Clinical presentation

Signs and symptoms are frequently non-specific and may include:

- Swinging pyrexia, wasting, and anorexia.
- Epigastric fullness and tenderness.
- Shoulder pain (referred due to irritation of the phrenic nerve).
- Persistent hiccups.

Imaging

Plain film

- *Erect CXR:* pneumoperitoneum or a pleural effusion, elevation or tenting of the diaphragm, basal consolidation on side of abscess.
- *Abdominal X-ray:* gas/fluid level adjacent to the diaphragm, an irregular pocket of gas or a soft tissue mass. Secondary paralytic ileus may also be seen.

Ultrasound (Fig. 23.20a)

Particularly valuable in detection of gas-free abscesses, also used to guide the insertion of a drain for treatment.

CT (Fig. 23.20b)

Allows identification of the abscess/assessment of the other abdominal organs or further collections. CT can also be used to guide drainage.

Information for the radiologist

History/details of any previous operations, dates of previous drainages, clotting result.

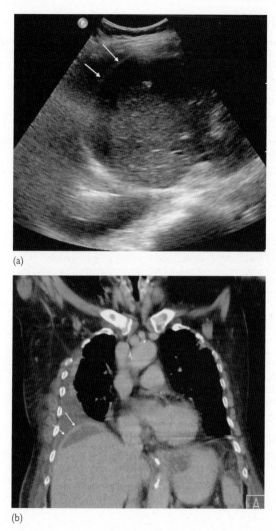

Fig. 23.20 a) Ultrasound image showing fluid collection overlying the liver, beneath the diaphragm (arrows). b) Coronal CT showing right-sided subphrenic abscess, seen as fluid attenuation below the diaphragm (arrows).

Diverticular disease

Diverticula develop when the mucosa herniates through points of weakness in the muscle layers of the colon wall at sites of vascular penetration.

- Diverticulosis = the presence of colonic diverticula.
- Diverticulitis = when inflammation is present.
- Sigmoid colon is the most common site. Only 15% of patients have right-sided diverticulosis.

Clinical presentation

Prevalence increases with age, although most remain asymptomatic. It is commonly an incidental finding. Causes include changes in colonic wall resistance, disordered motility, and reduced dietary fibre intake.

Imaging

- Role is to establish the diagnosis, severity, and extent.
- Confirm active inflammation in diverticulitis.
- Identify any complications—abscess, perforation, fistula formation, haemorrhage.

Fluoroscopy—barium enema

- Traditional test, CT, however, now often first line.
- Air/barium filled outpouchings extending from the lumen.
- Stricture length and calibre malignant stricture must be excluded.
  Features in favour of diverticular stricture include:
  - Stricture >10cm.
  - Intact mucosa.
  - Adjacent diverticula (may also coexist with tumour).
  - Smooth transition with normal colon cf. shouldered margins of malignant stricture ('apple core lesion').

CT (Fig. 23.21)

- Thickened bowel wall >3mm, with inflammation.
- Abscess formation: gas/fluid collection.
- Free intraperitoneal air/localized locules = perforation.
- Fistulation: 65% of colovesical fistulae occur as a result of diverticular disease (differential diagnosis is malignancy and Crohn's disease).
- CT angiography is used in active bleeding.

Information for the radiologist

Accurate clinical history, with attention to features suggesting bleeding, malignancy, fistula, etc. Sigmoidoscopy findings.

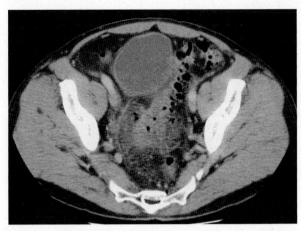

Fig. 23.21 Axial CT image showing a length of thickened sigmoid colon, with diverticulitis, pericolonic inflammatory change, and locules of pericolonic gas.

Volvulus

- Twisting of a segment of bowel with subsequent obstruction. The sigmoid colon and caecum are most commonly affected due to the long, mobile mesentery.
- Risk factors: increased age (caecal younger 30–60 years), chronic constipation, mental handicap, institutionalization.

Clinical presentation

- Sigmoid: lower abdominal pain and progressive abdominal distension, may be spontaneously relieved by passage of a large amount of flatus/faeces, may develop complete obstruction.
- Caecal: symptoms are those of acute bowel obstruction including pain, distension, and vomiting.

Treatment is with decompression via a rectal tube through the twisted segment (sigmoid), surgical resection of redundant loop sometimes required. Unrelieved obstruction may lead to bowel infarction/perforation.

Imaging

Plain film

- Sigmoid: bowel loop dilated to occupy the whole abdomen, with the appearance of an inverted 'U' (resembling a 'coffee bean'). Sigmoid loop typically devoid of haustra, with apex on the left of the abdomen. Remaining large bowel is often dilated, which is not seen in caecal volvulus.
- Caecal: caecum usually twists and inverts so the caecal pole occupies the left upper quadrant. The attached gas-filled appendix is sometimes seen. 1 or 2 haustral markings can still be seen. Often marked gaseous or fluid distension of small bowel. The left colon is usually collapsed.

CT

Performed when clinical and plain film assessment is inconclusive. As well as the signs previously described on plain film, the 'whirl sign' on CT reflects the twisted bowel and mesentery, along with demonstration of complications such as ischaemia and perforation.

Fluoroscopy

If diagnostic doubt, a water-soluble contrast enema can be performed (risk of perforation contraindicates the use of barium). Features at the point of torsion include a smooth, curved tapering of the colonic lumen to give a 'bird's beak appearance', although CT increasingly used as first line.

Information for the radiologist

- Presenting symptoms and signs, any clinical suspicion of ischaemia.

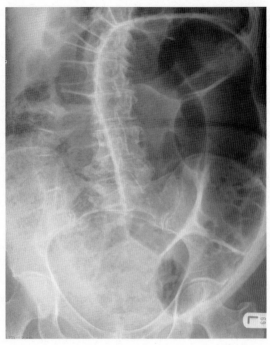

Fig. 23.22 Abdominal X-ray showing grossly dilated loop of large bowel within the left abdomen in a patient with sigmoid volvulus.

Intussusception

Intussusception is the telescoping, or prolapse of one part of bowel into an adjacent segment. The prolapsed segment is referred to as the intussusceptum and the receiving segment is the intussuscipiens. The most common sites are ileo–colic and ileo–ileo–colic.

Clinical presentation

Commonest in children 3 months–3 years. Majority are idiopathic with no lead point other than lymphoid hyperplasia. In adults 90% have a lead-point including lymphoma, polyps, tumours, Meckel's diverticulum, etc.

In children, presenting features are of intermittent colicky pain with drawing up of the legs with or without vomiting. The child may be completely well between episodes. Initially there may be watery stools but later the patient may pass blood and mucus in the classically described 'redcurrant jelly stools'. In late presentations, there may be features of bowel obstruction and shock, with possible ischaemia. In adults, abdominal pain, nausea and vomiting are common over weeks–months.

Imaging

Plain film

Abdominal X-ray normal in 50%. Classic findings include a soft tissue mass (most commonly in the right upper quadrant) and air crescent sign outlining the apex of the intussusceptum.

Ultrasound (Fig. 23.23a)

First-line investigation for intussusception. Free fluid is a common finding and does not preclude air enema.

CT (Fig. 23.23b)

In adults, CT is usually the first investigation, and may reveal the lead point.

Fluoroscopy

Single contrast/air enema demonstrates the obstruction, and reduction with air enema is the mainstay of treatment in uncomplicated paediatric intussusception. Air reduction should only be carried out in a centre with paediatric surgery and the child must be adequately resuscitated and haemodynamically stable. An NG tube is advised to decompress the stomach. Absolute contraindications are peritonism, perforation, or persisting shock. There is no role for this in adults.

Information for the radiologist

Predisposing conditions, duration of symptoms, and clinical condition of the patient.

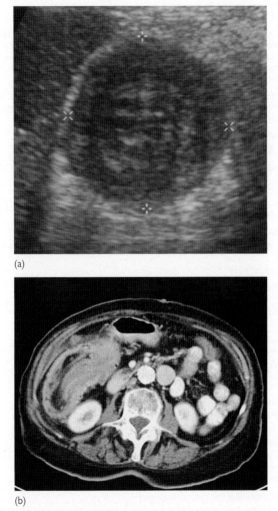

(a)

(b)

Fig. 23.23 a) Ultrasound image showing 'doughnut' appearance in a 2-year-old with intussusception. b) Axial CT showing intussuscepting loop of bowel within the right flank, giving the typical 'bowel within bowel' appearance.

Acute pancreatitis

Around 80% mild and self-limiting, 20% severe, associated with pancreatic necrosis and marked systemic response, may lead to multi organ failure. *Causes:* alcohol, gallstones, iatrogenic (post ERCP), drugs, trauma, metabolic e.g. increased Ca^{2+}, infection, congenital (pancreas divisum/annular pancreas), tumour, idiopathic.

Pathophysiology: unregulated activation of pancreatic enzymes leads to autodigestion of the gland causing inflammation and necrosis. Leakage of enzymes into the surrounding structures causes local complications.

Clinical presentation

Epigastric/central abdominal pain. Vomiting.

Imaging

- Confirm diagnosis and identify cause.
- Assess severity of pancreatitis, progression and complications.
- Guide interventional procedures, e.g. drainage of peripancreatic abscess.

Ultrasound

Detects gallstones. Pancreas often obscured by body habitus and bowel gas.

CT (Fig. 23.24)

Triple phase CT is the imaging modality of choice. CT <72 hours may not reflect the true severity of pancreatitis, only used if diagnostic doubt.

Mild

May be normal/mild enlargement/inflammation.

Severe

- Necrosis: non-enhancement of the gland.
- Peripancreatic fluid collections.
- Infection: may see locules of gas.
- Pseudocyst: collection of secretions.

Extra-pancreatic complications

- Pleural effusions, ascites, pseudoaneurysm of SMA/splenic artery, thrombosis SMV/splenic vein, secondary GI tract involvement.

MRI

Comparable to CT but CT usually more readily available/quicker test in ill patients. MRCP assesses integrity of the ducts as well as detect anatomical anomalies.

Information for the radiologist

Likely aetiology, how far into the disease process, clinical signs of sepsis, clotting if need for intervention.

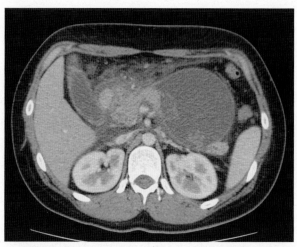

Fig. 23.24 Axial CT showing ill-defined inflammation of the pancreatic head, and a large fluid-collection occupying the body of the pancreas, in keeping with a pseudocyst.

Chronic pancreatitis

Irreversible, inflammatory fibrosis of the pancreas leading to endocrine and exocrine insufficiency.

Causes: alcohol (~70%), idiopathic (~20%), rarely: familial, cystic fibrosis, haemochromatosis, pancreatic duct obstruction, hyperparathyroidism, pancreas divisum.

Clinical presentation

Abdominal pain, normal/mildly elevated pancreatic enzymes; later diabetes mellitus and steatorrhoea.

Imaging

Imaging findings reflect parenchymal fibrosis, atrophy, duct strictures, and dilation with calcification.

Ultrasound

- Calcifications.
- Heterogeneous echo texture.
- Focal hypoechoic mass; difficult to distinguish from malignancy.
- Alternating strictures/dilatation of main pancreatic duct.
- Complications: pseudocysts, vascular complications (use Doppler).

EUS

Overcomes bowel gas and body fat which limits TA ultrasound. High-resolution images identify more subtle features including:

- Lobular outer margin of the gland.
- Prominent hyperechoic septa in the parenchyma due to fibrosis.
- Duct abnormalities: hyperechoic margins, ectasia of side branches, intraductal stones.

MRI/MRCP (Fig. 23.25)

In early chronic pancreatitis, signal intensity changes in keeping with fibrosis. In late chronic pancreatitis there is atrophy and pseudocyst formation. *MRCP* demonstrates ductal strictures and dilation, ectasia, sacculations, and intraductal stones (signal voids).

CT

- Dilated pancreatic duct and side branches.
- Calcifications: most specific CT finding.
- Atrophy (may be normal aging).
- Focal inflammatory mass/enlargement.
- Complications, e.g. pseudocyst, vascular complications.

Information for the radiologist

Any known risk factors, any clinical suspicion of malignancy.

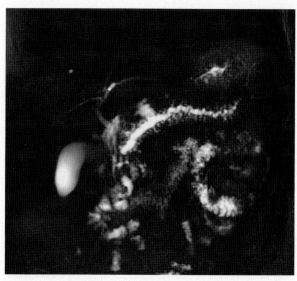

Fig. 23.25 Coronal MRCP image showing ectatic dilatation of the main pancreatic duct, with dilated side-branches, in keeping with chronic pancreatitis.

Cirrhosis

Characterized by diffuse parenchymal necrosis, regeneration, and scarring with abnormal reconstruction of pre-existing lobular architecture. The abnormal liver architecture interferes with the function and blood flow within the liver, which leads to portal hypertension.

Commonest cause in the West is alcohol, and viral infection (hepatitis) is the commonest worldwide cause.

Clinical presentation

Early symptoms are non-specific: anorexia, weakness, fatigue, weight loss, and pyrexia. In advanced disease patients may have signs of portal hypertension, such as ascites, bleeding from oesophageal varices, hepatic encephalopathy.

Imaging

Characteristic features are regenerating nodules separated by fibrous septae and loss of normal lobular architecture within the nodules. Nodular lesions may be regenerative nodules, dysplastic nodules or hepatocellular carcinoma (HCC).

Ultrasound

- Hepatomegaly with a nodular surface.
- Signs of fatty infiltration/coarsening of the liver texture.
- Signs of portal hypertension (ascites, splenomegaly), abnormal Doppler of hepatic artery/portal vein.
- Ultrasound-guided liver biopsy. (Transjugular biopsy can be performed if deranged uncorrectable clotting.)

CT (Fig. 23.26)

Finding similar to ultrasound. CT may be more sensitive identifying liver lesions.

MRI

Used as a problem-solving tool, to differentiate regenerative nodules from hepatocellular carcinoma.

Intervention

In severe portal hypertension a shunt between the portal and hepatic veins can be created to decrease pressure in the portal system: Transjugular intrahepatic portosystemic shunt (TIPSS) procedure.

Information for the radiologist

Aetiology of cirrhosis (if known), clinical symptoms (i.e. severity of suspected portal hypertension), clotting (if intervention is to be performed).

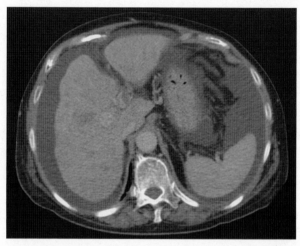

Fig. 23.26 Axial CT showing shrunken, nodular liver, ascites and dilated vessels adjacent to the stomach, in keeping with varices in a patient with alcoholic liver disease.

Ascites

This is the presence of fluid in the peritoneal cavity. In the supine position, ascitic fluid collects in the most dependent parts, initially around the liver, then in the pelvis and paracolic gutters.

Clinical presentation

There is fullness in the flanks with shifting dullness. Tense ascites is uncomfortable and may produce respiratory distress. A pleural effusion (usually right-sided) and peripheral oedema may be present.

Imaging

Plain film

There is generalized haziness of the abdomen with loss of the psoas outlines. Gas-containing small bowel loops float centrally.

Ultrasound (Fig. 23.27a)

This accurately localizes fluid in the abdomen and helps to estimate the degree of ascites. Fluid appears anechoic (dark), and bowel loops are usually seen floating freely within it. Ascitic fluid can be aspirated under ultrasound guidance for a diagnostic tap and the following examined:

• WCC.
• Gram stain and culture.
• Protein (transudate ≥11g/L; exudate <11g/L).
• Cytology for malignant cells.
• Amylase to exclude pancreatic ascites.

Percutaneous drainage by means of a catheter can also be performed under ultrasound guidance where indicated.

Further indication for ultrasound is in the examination of the abdomen and pelvis for a possible cause of ascites, such as cirrhosis or malignancy, with clinical guidance as to the most likely suspected cause.

CT (Fig. 23.27b)

This demonstrates ascites as a low density margin around the intra-abdominal organs. The attenuation values of ascites range from 0 to +30 HU. CT attenuation values increase with increasing protein content as a general rule. Haemorrhagic ascites can be identified by its higher attenuation value (>30HU).

Information for the radiologist

• Underlying cause (if known).
• INR—should not have been obtained >24 hours prior to any planned ascitic tap or drain insertion.

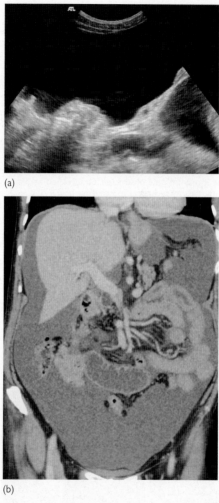

(a)

(b)

Fig. 23.27 a) Ultrasound image of the abdomen in a patient with liver disease showing free intraperitoneal fluid. b) Coronal CT from a different patient showing widespread intra-abdominal fluid, secondary to primary peritoneal carcinomatosis.

Hernia

The protrusion of a viscus/part of a viscus from the cavity in which it is normally contained. Most hernia occur in the abdomen. Hernias are irreducible if they cannot be pushed back into the right place. Incarcerated hernias are no longer reducible. Obstruction means that bowel contents can't pass through the hernia. Strangulated hernia occur when the vascular supply is compromised.

Inguinal: commonest type, men >women. For a full list of hernia types, see 📖 *OHCM*, p614.

Clinical presentation

Generally asymptomatic—may complain of a fullness at the hernia site, aching, or the lump may enlarge on increasing intra-abdominal pressure/standing.

If the hernia becomes incarcerated, there may be enlargement of the hernia, and it may become obstructed. Strangulated hernia may present with systemic toxicity secondary to ischaemic bowel.

Imaging

Plain film

An inguinal hernia may be identified, but this isn't sensitive or specific. Useful if present with a small bowel obstruction.

Ultrasound

Increasingly used in the outpatient investigation of groin pain to confirm the presence of a groin hernia if equivocal examination. This has replaced herniography.

CT

May be helpful to diagnose spigelian or obturator hernia, or if unable to examine the patient due to body habitus, and ultrasound failed.

Information for the radiologist

Any signs of ischaemic compromise clinically.

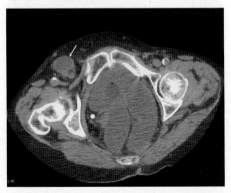

Fig. 23.28 Axial CT scan showing dilated loops of fluid-filled obstructed small bowel, secondary to a right-sided groin hernia (arrow).

Breast differential diagnosis

Gynaecomastia

Abnormal amount of breast tissue in men.
- Physiological.
- Drugs:
  - Oestrogen, anti-androgens, etc.
- Pathological:
  - Hypogonadism.
  - Cirrhosis.
  - Hyperthyroidism.
  - Tumours: oestrogen producing, e.g. testicular; HCG producing, e.g. testicular, bronchial cancers.

Solitary lesion at mammography

Malignant:
- Carcinoma.
- Phyllodes tumour.

Benign:
- Cyst.
- Fibroadenoma.
- Intramammary lymph node.
- Galactocoele.
- Papilloma.
- Abscess.

Multiple lesions at mammography

- Cysts.
- Fibroadenomas.
- Skin lesions, e.g. neurofibromas.
- Intramammary lymph nodes.
- Metastases.

Breast conditions

Mammography

A mammogram is an X-ray examination of the breast. It is a highly effective imaging method for detecting, diagnosing, and managing a variety of breast diseases, especially cancer.

Indications

1. Evaluation of breast symptoms as part of triple assessment

Females may present with symptoms such as a breast lump, pain, nipple thickening or discharge, skin or nipple retraction, or a change in breast size and shape. Symptomatic females have a mammogram and ultrasound as appropriate depending on the clinical presentation. However, young women have higher breast parenchymal density, making it difficult to differentiate between tumour and normal breast tissue on mammography. Ultrasound is more sensitive than mammography in young women and is the first-line investigation in women aged <35 years.

Triple assessment involves clinical examination, imaging (mammography and ultrasound), and pathology. All components of triple assessment are graded 1 to 5: 1 = normal, 2 = benign, 3 = indeterminate, 4 = suspicious, 5 = malignant. Any discordance between the three arms of triple assessment requires further investigation. For example, a palpable lump that is suspicious on clinical examination but has no correlate on imaging still requires clinical core biopsy to secure a histological diagnosis. It is always the arm with the highest suspicion that drives further management.

2. Surveillance following breast cancer surgery

Annual mammograms are performed for 5–10 years following surgery for breast cancer. The duration of follow-up is influenced by local policies and the patient's individual risk taking into account factors such as tumour size and axillary node involvement.

3. NHS Breast Screening Programme

UK population screening started in 1988. The screening programme has been shown to reduce mortality from breast cancer by 30%. Asymptomatic women aged 50–70 years are invited for 3-yearly mammograms. By 2012, the screening programme will be extended to include women aged 47–73 years.

4. Family history surveillance

Annual or 18-monthly mammograms are performed in women with moderate to very high risk of breast cancer. MRI will also be performed in the very high-risk group.

Technique

Two views of each breast are obtained, a mediolateral oblique (MLO) view and a craniocaudal (CC) view (Fig. 25.1). The breast is compressed between two plates so that the maximum amount of tissue can be imaged with minimum X-ray dose. Both analogue and digital mammography are available. Analogue mammography utilizes film as both a receptor and a display for the image, producing static, fixed images. However, digital mammography uses detectors that change the X-rays into electrical signals. These signals are then transferred to a digital receptor that converts the X-ray energy to numbers, processes the numbers, and produces an image that can be displayed on a monitor. The main advantage of digital mammography is the opportunity to manipulate and further optimize image quality following the original acquisition.

Dose

The accepted measure of dose in mammography is the mean glandular dose, which is the average dose to the glandular tissue of the breast. It is expressed in unit of milligray (mGy). The radiation dose for a standard two-view examination is approximately 4.5mGy. This is equivalent to a few months of natural background radiation. A risk:benefit calculation has established that the benefits of screening far outweigh the risk of inducing a cancer, with the ratio of lives saved to lives lost calculated as approximately 100:1.

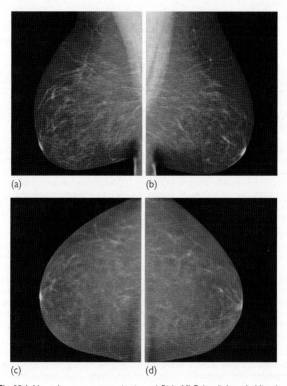

(a) (b)

(c) (d)

Fig. 25.1 Normal mammogram projections. a) Right MLO (mediolateral oblique). b) Left MLO. c) Right craniocaudal (CC). d) Left CC.

Breast cancer

Breast cancer is the most common cancer in the UK. The lifetime risk of developing breast cancer is 1 in 9 for women and 1 in 1014 for men. The majority of invasive breast cancers are adenocarcinomas (85% ductal, 15% lobular). The main risk factors are increasing age, personal history of breast cancer, previous breast biopsies demonstrating atypia, positive family history, early menarche, late menopause, and nulliparity.

Clinical presentation

Females usually present with a painless palpable lump which is often firm or irregular. Nipple changes (inversion, discharge, eczema) and skin changes (tethering, peau d'orange) can also occur.

Imaging

Mammography

Invasive carcinomas typically appear as an ill-defined, spiculate mass causing architectural distortion (Fig. 25.2). Non-invasive carcinomas typically present as pleomorphic segmental microcalcification.

Ultrasound

Targeted breast ultrasound helps to further characterize the mass. Classically a carcinoma is seen as an irregular, hypoechoic mass with posterior acoustic shadowing (Fig. 25.3). The tumour tends to be taller than it is wide as it disrupts tissue planes. Colour Doppler imaging demonstrates abnormal vascularity with centrally penetrating vessels.

Ultrasound of the axilla is performed for local staging. Features concerning for malignant infiltration of lymph nodes include a short axis diameter of >5mm, thickened cortex >2mm, or complete loss of the central fatty hilum. Lymph nodes with malignant or suspicious features require fine needle aspiration cytology. If the lymph nodes are confirmed to be positive for metastatic disease on cytology, the patient will undergo axillary clearance. If the nodes are negative, then the patient will have sentinel node biopsy at the time of surgery.

MRI

Contrast-enhanced MRI highlights neovascularity in malignant lesions that demonstrate rapid uptake and washout of contrast. It is utilized selectively to aid local staging in patients who have tumours that are difficult to accurately size both clinically and with routine imaging. In particular, lobular carcinoma has a propensity for multifocality and defining the true extent of disease is vital. If the tumour proves too large for breast conserving surgery (wide local excision), then a mastectomy is necessary. In addition, MRI is used to assess the response to neoadjuvant chemotherapy and the detection of recurrence in the post-surgical breast.

CT

Complete staging with CT of the thorax, abdomen, and pelvis is performed in patients with malignant involvement of the axillary lymph nodes or features suspicious for metastatic spread.

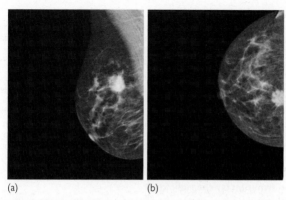

(a)   (b)

Fig. 25.2 a) and b) Spiculate mass seen in the 12 o'clock position of the right breast.

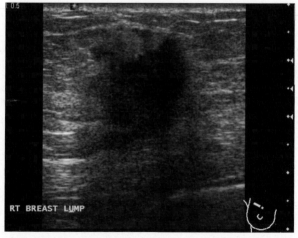

Fig. 25.3 Ultrasound image demonstrating an irregular hypoechoic mass at the 12 o'clock position of the right breast, with extensive posterior shadowing.

Bone scan

Bone metastases are the most common site of distant spread in breast cancer. Bone scan is used routinely in patients with involved axillary nodes or with bone pain.

Image-guided biopsy

All indeterminate to malignant lesions in the breast require needle core biopsy for histological confirmation. This can be performed clinically but increasingly biopsies are done under imaging control because this is more accurate. If the mass can be localized with ultrasound, this is the preferred imaging modality as it is the quickest technique with real-time visualization of the needle sampling the mass. However, if the lesion can only be seen with mammography, then X-ray-guided biopsy is utilized. MRI-guided biopsy is performed if the mass is occult on both mammography and ultrasound. This technique is only available in specialist centres and is very time consuming.

Information for the radiologist

Relevant risk factors including the patient's age, personal history of breast cancer and positive family history. The clinical score (P1 = normal, P2 = benign, P3 = indeterminate, P4 = suspicious for malignancy, P5 = malignant) is vital to ensure appropriate correlation with imaging findings. The presence of chronic kidney disease (GFR <30ml/min) is significant as this may preclude giving iodinated (CT) or gadolinium based (MR) contrast.

Breast abscess

A breast abscess is a localized collection of pus, usually in a periareolar location. Breast infections are fairly common, particularly during breast-feeding. The nipple and areola can become dry and chapped, with suckling causing cracks in the skin through which bacteria can infiltrate. The most common organism is *Staphylococcus aureus*. Older women, particularly smokers can present with recurrent periareolar sepsis related to duct ectasia which is benign dilatation of the main subareolar milk ducts.

Clinical presentation

Presenting features include pain associated with a localized area of erythema and induration. In later stages, there may be a tender, fluctuant mass representing the abscess. Systemic features include pyrexia, tachycardia, and vomiting. The appearance of the skin is similar to what can be seen with an inflammatory cancer. However, an infective process is typically painful, while an inflammatory cancer rarely is. If there is a high clinical suspicion for malignancy or the patient fails to respond to therapy, a biopsy should be performed.

Imaging

A breast abscess is usually managed clinically and treated conservatively with antibiotics. Imaging is not required unless the patient fails to respond to therapy.

Mammography

It is not used in the acute phase because it is extremely painful. Mammography should be performed in women >35 years of age once the acute infection has resolved to rule out an underlying malignancy.

Ultrasound

The skin appears thickened with pockets of fluid between the skin and subcutaneous tissue consistent with oedema. An abscess can have a varied appearance (Fig. 25.4). At one end of the spectrum, it can appear cystic in nature with low level internal echoes. In certain cases, it can appear more complex resembling a solid, hypoechoic mass. If the infectious process does not resolve with antibiotics, then ultrasound-guided aspiration of the abscess is helpful.

Information for the radiologist

Is the patient currently breastfeeding? If they have been treated with antibiotics, has there been a positive response? If not, is ultrasound guided aspiration required? The clinical score (P1 = normal, P2 = benign, P3 = indeterminate, P4 = suspicious for malignancy, P5 = malignant) is vital to ensure appropriate correlation with imaging findings.

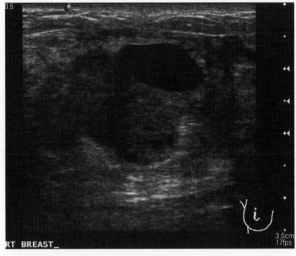

Fig. 25.4 Ultrasound image demonstrating a mixed solid/cystic lesion consistent with an abscess.

Breast cyst

Cysts arise in the terminal ductal lobular unit as a result of an imbalance between the production and resorption of secretions. Often, cysts are multiple and bilateral. Cysts are common in the perimenopausal years, with a peak incidence between the ages of 40 and 50 years. In younger lactating females, the cysts may be filled with milk and termed a galactocoele. Simple cysts are not associated with malignancy.

Clinical presentation

One or several palpable smooth, fluctuant, benign feeling lumps. Occasionally, a tense cyst can present as a discrete hard mass.

Imaging

Mammography

A cyst appears as a well-defined, round or oval mass (Fig. 25.5). Sometimes a thin lucent halo is seen surrounding the mass. Occasionally, fine curvilinear 'eggshell' calcification is seen in the cyst wall. A galactocoele that has sufficient fat content may be visible as a radiolucent mass or even demonstrate a fat-fluid level in upright lateral mammograms. These features are not specific and ultrasound imaging is necessary to evaluate if the mass is solid or a fluid-filled cyst.

Ultrasound

A simple cyst has well-defined margin (Fig. 25.6). It has no internal echoes and there is increased through transmission of the ultrasound beam reflecting its fluid content. A galactocoele can look like a simple cyst or occasionally have low level internal echoes due to the fat content (Fig. 25.7). Features of a complex cyst include the presence of internal echoes, thin septations or a thickened irregular wall. A cyst may be aspirated if the patient is symptomatic or if there is any diagnostic uncertainty. Fluid is sent for cytology only if blood-stained or if there are atypical sonographic features.

Information for the radiologist

It is useful to document if lactating. Relevant risk factors including the patient's age, personal history of breast cancer, and positive family history. The clinical score (P1 = normal, P2 = benign, P3 = indeterminate, P4 = suspicious for malignancy, P5 = malignant) is vital to ensure appropriate correlation with imaging findings.

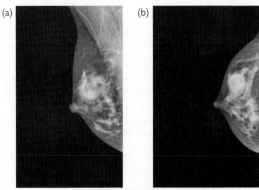

Fig. 25.5 a) MLO projection and b) CC projections of the right breast demonstrating a well-defined mass in the upper outer quadrant of the right breast.

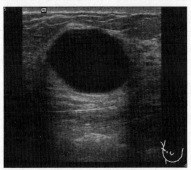

Fig. 25.6 Ultrasound demonstrating a well-defined simple cyst with posterior acoustic enhancement.

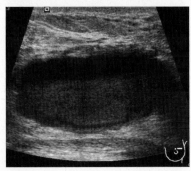

Fig. 25.7 Ultrasound demonstrating thick walled cyst with internal echoes in keeping with a galactocoele.

Fibroadenoma

A fibroadenoma is the result of idiopathic overgowth of the specialized stromal connective tissue within the breast lobule. It is the most common cause of a benign solid mass in the breast. In the majority of cases they are solitary, but in 20% of females they can be multiple. Fibroadenomas are hormone sensitive and tend to increase in size during pregnancy and involute in the perimenopausal period. Peak incidence is in the 3rd decade.

Clinical presentation

Fibroadenomas present clinically as a smooth, firm, mobile mass. It is sometimes referred to as a 'breast mouse' because of its mobility within the breast tissue.

Imaging

Mammography

A fibroadenoma is seen as a well-circumscribed, oval mass. Sometimes a thin, lucent halo is seen surrounding the mass. In older women, as the fibroadenoma involutes, coarse 'popcorn' calcification may be seen associated with the mass.

Ultrasound

It is seen as a well-defined, ovoid, hypoechoic mass with a thin echogenic pseudocapsule (Fig. 25.8). As the tumour grows along tissue planes, it tends to be wider than it is tall. Despite sonographic features consistent with benign disease, needle core biopsy for histological diagnosis is performed either clinically or under direct vision with ultrasound guidance. This is necessary to ensure that well-circumscribed cancers are not missed. Once a benign histological diagnosis is obtained, no further intervention is required.

Information for the radiologist

Relevant risk factors including the patient's age, personal history of breast cancer, and positive family history. The clinical score (P1 = normal, P2 = benign, P3 = indeterminate, P4 = suspicious for malignancy, P5 = malignant) is vital to ensure appropriate correlation with imaging findings.

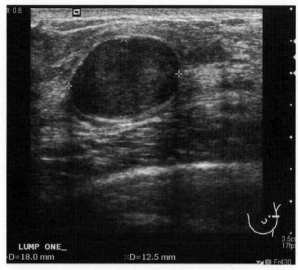

Fig. 25.8 Ultrasound demonstrating a well-defined solid hypoechoic mass with a thin echogenic capsule in keeping with a fibroadenoma.

Papilloma

A papilloma is a tumour that arises in a duct, either centrally or peripherally within the breast. It represents a focal proliferation of the ductal epithelium that projects into the lumen of the duct. Papillomas are largely considered benign lesions, especially if solitary within a large subareolar duct. Multiple papillomas tend to be within smaller, peripheral ducts and are associated with an increased likelihood of atypia and malignancy.

Clinical presentation

Papillomas are associated with overproduction of secretions that are not balanced by the normal resorptive mechanisms of the duct. This results in distension of the duct and nipple discharge. As they are friable structures that bleed easily, the nipple discharge may be blood-stained. Occasionally, a palpable mass is evident.

Imaging

Mammography

Papillomas are often not appreciated on mammography due to their small size and intraductal location. When imaging findings are present, they include a well-circumscribed subareolar mass, solitary or multiple dilated ducts, and infrequently a cluster of microcalcifications.

Ultrasound

Characteristically, papillomas appear as a hypoechoic, lobulated mass within a dilated duct or cyst (Figs. 25.9 and 25.10). Due to the association with malignancy, needle core biopsy under ultrasound guidance is performed for histological diagnosis. If there are no features of atypia, it can be removed percutaneously with a vacuum-assisted biopsy device. If there are features of atypia, then surgical excision is necessary.

Information for the radiologist

If there is nipple discharge, is it blood-stained? Relevant risk factors including the patient's age, personal history of breast cancer, and positive family history. If there is a palpable mass, the clinical score (P1 = normal, P2 = benign, P3 = indeterminate, P4 = suspicious for malignancy, P5 = malignant) is vital to ensure appropriate correlation with imaging findings.

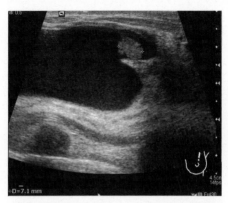

Fig. 25.9 Ultrasound image demonstrating 7mm solid papilloma seen projecting into the lumen of the cyst.

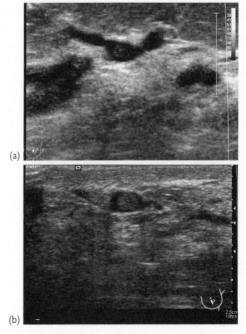

Fig. 25.10 a) and b) Ultrasound images demonstrating 6mm papilloma seen sitting within a dilated duct.

Index